The *Imperfect* Vegan

Making a difference on a
(mostly) plant-based diet

CAT WHITE

Copyright ©2023 Catherine Elizabeth White

All rights reserved.

ISBN (print) 978-0-6459335-0-5
ISBN (e-book) 978-0-6459335-2-9

No portion of this book may be reproduced in any form without written permission from the publisher or author, except as permitted by Australian copyright law, or small sections quoted in a review.

Before putting any of the concepts, ideas, habits, and ways of living into practice, please bear in mind that I am not a health professional. *The Imperfect Vegan* is based on my own opinions, observations, and careful research, but it should not be considered a substitute for the advice of a qualified doctor or health practitioner. Always seek professional medical advice before adopting any of the ideas suggested in this book into your own health regimen, as I and my publisher disclaim responsibility for any adverse effects that may arise from the use of any material contained within it. While I have strived for balance, fairness, and factuality as of the time of publication, please consider the thoughts presented here as my own personal experience and opinion. Information is correct at the time of publishing.

Cover Design: Steph Webber marmelocreative.com

Editor: Rob Peace robpeaceliterary.com

Formatting: Tonia Nazzaro mstoniadesigns.com

First print and e-book edition 2023.

www.catwhite.net

To Bel,
Without you, the seed of this book would not have been planted.

and

To Phil,
My favourite meat eater. I love us.

Contents

Introduction	1
Part 1: What's So Wrong with the Animal Industry?	17
Chapter 1: Climate Change	19
Chapter 2: Exploitation	52
Chapter 3: Marketing and Myths	74
Part 2: Letting Go of Perfection	135
Chapter 4: There's No Such Thing as a Perfect Vegan	137
Chapter 5: Why It's So Hard	145
Chapter 6: Being Human	163
Part 3: What You Can Do	174
Chapter 7: We Need to Do Something	176
Chapter 8: Get Educated	194
Chapter 9: Allow the Transition	212
Chapter 10: Connect with Support	226
Chapter 11: Be the Lighthouse	240
Final Words: Making a Difference	246
What's Next?	259
Acknowledgements	260
Helpful Resources	263
References	269

INTRODUCTION

I'd consider it fair to say that I'm not your typical vegan. Of course, you likely gathered that from the title of this book, in which I confess my flaws (or 'imperfections') right off the proverbial bat. But I have nothing to hide. Why write a book unless I'm going to be completely transparent? So let's just get this out of the way before we go any further:

I'm not much of an animal lover.

I know. Kind of a strange thing for a vegan to say. But let me try and redeem myself before you toss this book into the bin.

For certain, I think that animals are awesome creatures. And I'm happy that they exist—even spiders. We need all of them, as they contribute to our diverse ecosystem that supports life on our planet. They also have the right to exist 'just because'—that's definitely not in question. I just don't get all doe-eyed looking at a cow or a bird or a fluffy chicken. Or even a doe. But, of course, I certainly wish them no harm, and they should be able to live their lives free from human exploitation. I also acknowledge that what we do to them in factory farms, slaughterhouses, and research laboratories is abhorrent, and I want no part of it by giving my money to the companies responsible for those things.

While I know this intellectually, and it tugs at my heartstrings whenever watching or reading about it, I must admit I don't feel an enduring emotional connection. Suffice to say that it wasn't the painful plight of animals that got me into veganism.

It wasn't for health reasons, either. While I *do* want to eat well and be as healthy as possible, diet doesn't drive me, nor do I have a disease to manage. I've long known the benefits of eating whole foods, so it wasn't much of a leap to cut out animal products and add more plants. And while I'm conscious that chickens are full of 'faecal soup', fish are riddled with microplastics, and chocolate is chockful of sugar, I still succumb to cravings for food that I'm well aware is not good for me.

So then…why veganism? Like a growing number of people, I turned to this way of eating for the environmental impact. Simple mathematics reveal that there's not enough land to feed all the people in the world the way we're currently doing, let alone with the ten billion people we're projected to have in only a couple of decades. For me, it's just common sense that I do my bit by eating more plants—not only to stem the tide, but to get used to it before significant change is

Introduction

inevitably thrust upon all of us. 'Vegan for the environment' makes sense to me logically, but I also have an emotional connection: I really don't want to end up a climate migrant, living off the land and fighting for survival. I like my house and my car and the internet; I like going to the cinema and the café around the corner and having convenient access to the shops for anything I may need at any time. And I'm sure I'm not alone—this book is your permission to admit it, too. Go on. I won't tell anyone.

When we look at the various reasons people choose to make food choices, deciding to get healthy or to manage disease with diet is a very personal journey, but it doesn't make the world any more or less habitable. Treating animals with moral consideration is important and worthwhile—I'm not here to deny that—but it won't affect our weather patterns whether it happens today or in a thousand years from now. Yet from an environmental perspective, what I choose to put on my plate *does* have a global impact. It's unfortunately not an understatement to say the very future of our species is at risk.

The United Nations has been advising the world to switch to a plant-based diet since 2006[1]—nearly 20 years ago. That's nearly as long ago as the final episode of Friends. And, also for decades now, climate scientists have been warning that by 2030 we'll be experiencing water wars, climate migration, and rising sea levels unless we limit our global temperature rise to under 1.5°C. The world has already warmed 1.1° compared to pre-industrial levels, with nine of the hottest years on record having been in the last decade[2]. Many countries have even breached 1.5°, including China, Italy, Brazil, Turkey, and Saudi Arabia. Others like Japan, Spain, and the mid-west USA have hit 1.4°, and some northern parts of Canada, Russia, and Scandinavia have even risen above 2.3°[3]. The evidence is irrefutable. The year 2030 is just around the corner, and we're starting to see the effects already[3-5].

Rising global temperatures doesn't only mean 'hot': it also means 'unstable'. I'm sure you've noticed more extreme weather events where you live, whether in the form of fires, droughts, floods, king tides, heatwaves, monsoonal rainfall, unseasonal snow, more frequent tornados…you get the ominous picture. However, for most of us in the Western world, we don't notice the worst of climate change yet because we still have the infrastructure to cope with it. We have emergency services, early warning systems, good drainage, and multiple access points to food and freshwater.

But as sea levels rise, we'll lose our coastal cities and have to migrate inland. Shipping ports will be flooded and global transport disrupted; we won't be able to move food around the world, let alone refuel our gas stations or import the latest smartphone. Power grids will go offline, meaning no hot water, no internet, and no global news stories. And amid all the disruption, we'll have to hunt and gather our own food (probably animals, seeing as we're in survival mode) and deal with crazy weather without roofs over our heads, and also devoid of things we take for granted like hospitals, rubbish collection, and Google Maps.

Hold up for a moment, though—let's take a step back: what's this got to do with being vegan? Well, according to many respected sources and scientists, the animal agriculture industry is a major contributor to climate change[1,6,7]. We'll examine this further in Part 1 of this book, but to introduce the

Introduction

topic, our climate is changing because we're trapping too much carbon dioxide (CO_2) in our atmosphere. Animal agriculture is the second largest contributor to CO_2 after oil and gas. It's even more than the entire global transport industry—that's all the trucks, planes, cars, and ships combined.

The more I've dug into this issue, the more I've found how the animal industry touches *everything*[8]. It's the leading cause of deforestation in the Amazon rainforest[9] and the largest driver of biodiversity loss on land[10] and in the ocean[11]. It's a leading contributor of ocean dead zones and water pollution[12,13], as well as the primary cause of plastics in the Great Pacific Garbage Patch[14]. Animal farming is a major source of land and water degradation, using 20% of our global freshwater supply just to grow the crops that feed its animals[15,16] (which, incidentally, is 750 times the amount needed to quench the annual thirst of every human on the planet). The practice occupies 80% of arable land and provides only 18% of our global calories[17]. Aside from the environmental impacts of this inefficient system that generates *less* output than the resources it inputs, there are also the issues of animal exploitation, human rights violations[18], zoonotic diseases (viruses that can jump from animals to humans, such as SARS and COVID)[19], and government lobbying[20].

How has the global animal agriculture system become such a huge issue? Partly because there's more people on the planet than ever, but mostly because no one (until now) has run the numbers to figure out if it's sustainable (it's not). But it's also because of our inflated demand for animal products. We as a species never used to eat this much meat or drink this much milk. Since the 1950s, our increased demand has been driven by clever marketing, governments releasing industry-influenced dietary guidelines, and subsidies provided for animal farmers to keep prices artificially low.

Although there are more reasons for being vegan than protecting the environment—not to mention the fact that being vegan is not the only thing that will solve climate change—addressing what we eat undeniably has a positive impact on many dire issues in our world.

You may have asked yourself, 'But *really*—how much of an impact can my individual choices make in the huge world?' Well, consider this: the only reason any company exists is because of the choices we consumers make regarding the food on our plate and the products in our shopping cart. If every single person in the world truly believed that their choices didn't affect anything at large, can you imagine the chaos? Things add up. They compound. A single, burning ember doesn't seem like anything to worry about, but if every house on the street had one of those embers simmering and smouldering away, the whole neighbourhood would be aflame in no time. Feel free to concoct your own less-fiery analogy—the point is that we're all global citizens, and our actions *do* impact those around us, even if that impact isn't immediately apparent.

While it may seem like a simple decision to cut out animal products and stop supporting these industries, the solution is not as straightforward. It's not always easy to choose consumer goods with no animal products, because they're ubiquitous. They're in almost *everything*. It's hard to change habits and tastebuds that have developed over a lifetime. It takes time to do research to find out where our food comes from and

Introduction

the impact of its production. The good news, however, is that we don't need to be perfect at this to still make a difference in the world: we can be imperfect vegans—if we choose to.

Should we choose to? At the end of the day, it's always your choice, and even after you've read my (hopefully, very) convincing argument in this book, you're free to make up your own mind with no judgement from me.

~

At this point, though, it's a good idea to define what exactly I mean by 'imperfect vegan'. Officially, veganism is a lifestyle (not just a diet) against 'all forms of exploitation of, and cruelty to, animals'[21], but as more people enter into veganism for different reasons, it takes on a wider, more inclusive definition.

While I've accidentally (all right, fine—maybe on purpose) instigated some very heated debates on social media by using the term 'part-time vegan', what I really mean is that whatever you can do towards the goals of veganism *is* going to make a difference in the world. An individual following a standard Western diet incorporating a program like Meat Free Mondays would save approximately 51 animals and 212,000 litres of water per year[22], which is equivalent to a diet with zero food miles[23]. Skipping just one cheeseburger saves enough water to go three months of brushing your teeth without turning off the tap (twice a day, of course). Even ordering a vegan meal just once at a restaurant demonstrates the demand for the product and encourages them to keep offering it.

Technically, what I'm advocating for could be called more well-known names like *vegetarian, flexitarian, climatarian,* or *plant-based*, but what do those actually mean? *Vegetarian* isn't enough, as dairy products can be some of the most environmentally damaging of all. *Flexitarian* is just wishy-washy and can mean basically anything, so you'd have to spend hours explaining your particular variation to anyone who asked. *Climatarian* is a new term, and while it addresses the need to be aware of the environment, it doesn't call out the explicit need to avoid or reduce animal products. It makes it seem like sustainability and locally sourced foods are the most important factor, which, as we'll see in Part 1 (spoiler alert) don't make a difference when the diet still includes animal products. *Plant-based* tends to refer only to diet, whereas the environmental damage can also come from animal exploitation in areas like entertainment, clothing, and other consumer goods.

For simplicity throughout this book, I'll use the term 'vegan', as it's the most commonly understood term. When we go to restaurants, we ask for the vegan menu. At shops, we check if the leather is vegan or if the nail polish is a vegan brand. And when I order the eggplant parmigiana at a restaurant and someone says, 'Are you vegan?', I just say yes.

I tend to use 'vegan' and 'plant-based' interchangeably, and although I encourage you to adopt whichever term you're most comfortable with, I also want you to know that my use of the term 'vegan' does not intend to diminish its original meaning. I believe that the more inclusive we make the vegan community, the more people will make vegan (or plant-based or climatarian or whatever word you choose) their default way of life, and the closer we'll come as a society to accomplishing the original mission. While vegan is the goal,

Introduction

I hold no expectations that you'll be perfect at it, and simply encourage you to be 'as vegan as you can', so to speak, in whatever way is best for you.

Hardcore vegans might say there's no such thing as 'mostly' vegan: you either are or you aren't. Sort of like, 'You can't be a little bit pregnant.' Being vegan is a point of moral consideration. And while I absolutely agree with the worthiness of the cause, it's not so black and white in practice. We're humans—not robots. Most of us have spent decades mindlessly eating the mainstream diet without considering where it comes from or what effect it has on our home, our planet. We've been influenced by clever marketing and societal norms, and we have powerful subconscious psychological behaviours that make it hard for us to change. This is normal, and we'll expand on this in Part 2.

An imperfect vegan is someone doing the best they can with what they know. It's someone who knows that life is a balancing act, full of conflicting priorities. They know that smaller changes—ones that fit with their lifestyle—are more sustainable over the long term. They know that they're making a difference, even if they're only making tiny changes.

~

Early on in my vegan journey, I was lamenting to a friend how hard it is to be vegan. *Animal products are in everything, I still have cravings for my old food, I don't know all the vegan alternatives, too many beans make me…you know…*

Then she said something that was an absolute game changer:

The Imperfect Vegan

'The world doesn't need 100 perfect vegans; the world needs billions of people doing the best they can.'

It helped me release the pressure on myself (pun absolutely intended), but it also helped me remember to celebrate the people in my life who are doing the best they can—even if that's simply supporting my choices without giving me a hard time.

It also planted the seed that eventually grew to be this book. My mission in life is not only to be the best vegan I can be (read that again: not the best vegan in the world, but the best vegan I'm capable of being), it's to inspire an enormous amount of people to reduce their demand on the animal industry. I believe that a mass movement in which *most* people choose plants *most* of the time is the best way to get us to a place in which we finally see the damaging effects of the animal industry disappear. There are many facets to this fight: we need political change, industry regulations, dietary education, support for animal farmers as they transition to plant products, great tasting plant-based alternatives to our favourite foods—as well as money for all these things—but the main catalyst that will get the wheels turning is consumer demand. Even if governments around the world ban animal farming outright, underground markets would soon spring up to meet the demand—just as they did with alcohol during the Prohibition era. As long as we're buying their products, they'll keep making them.

Today, it's never been easier to be vegan, and we're coming to the tipping point. The year 2021 saw record financial investments into dairy and meat alternatives, with $5 billion USD being pledged by investors[24]. And it's not only billionaires like Bill Gates, Jeff Bezos, and Richard Branson: dozens of

Introduction

traditional meat companies are also getting in on the plant-based protein action, including Tyson Foods, Nestlé, and Unilever[25,26].

The rise of plant-based fast-food chains, vegan cosmetics, and meat alternatives has made dietary change more accessible and acceptable to the mainstream consumer. In the US, sales of plant-based meats doubled between 2017 and 2021[27]. Overall, plant-based menu items in restaurants have grown a whopping 2,800% since 2018, and supermarket sales of plant-based items are growing at three times the rates of other foods. In 2022, oat milk sales grew by 22%, and plant milks now account for around 16% of the total milk market. Many cosmetic brands have converted to vegan products or pledged to be 100% cruelty-free in the coming years[28–32].

Vegan promotion is becoming more visible, too. In New York, public schools now have Plant Powered Fridays, where the main meal is vegan[33] and all NYC public hospitals serve plant-based meals as the default option for inpatients[34]. In Amsterdam, government events are catered as vegetarian by default, with meat or fish needing to be specifically requested in advance[35]. Taiwan has made it a legal requirement for governments to promote low-carbon diets, specifically plant-based foods[36]. New York City, Portland, and Las Vegas have Vegan Dining Month every January[37], which coincides with Veganuary, the worldwide program that challenges people to try veganism for a month.

In 2023, Veganuary celebrated its tenth anniversary with a record-breaking sign-up rate. More than 700,000 people participated, from every country on the globe except for two (Vatican City and North Korea, somewhat predictably on both counts), with a 75% increase in corporate participation and more than 1,500 new menu item listings[38]. As a society, we're becoming more aware of our impact on the climate, with a majority of shoppers saying they consider sustainability when making food choices. And through documentaries, reporting, and popular vegan celebrities, the façade of the meat industry is fading, and the invisibility it relies on so heavily is becoming exposed[39]. More and more people are identifying as vegan or at least flexitarian.

However, we're still pushing the boulder up the hill.

I really believe that once we reach the tipping point—when the boulder goes over the crest and starts rolling downhill under its own motion—plant-based choices will become the default, and it will be easier for everyone to choose vegan options. This will make it more likely that we'll achieve *all* goals—be they eliminating animal exploitation, preventing disease, or reversing climate change. We need as many people as possible, doing anything and everything they can to help push that boulder.

~

In a nutshell (the contents of which would be celebrated by vegans far and wide), that's why I wrote this book. I would honestly love to be wrong—please, *please* prove me wrong, actually—but the science is sadly pointing towards the problem. Thankfully, though, it's also pointing to the solution. We may not be able to solve everything ourselves, and the animal agriculture industry is certainly not the only thing that needs to be addressed, but reducing demand on animal products is

Introduction

the simplest, quickest, and most powerful impact an individual can make on their own. Working together, collective action is more powerful than government intervention. Not only is this the best option for our planet, but it also happens to be the most optimal for our personal health, and the kindest choice for all other sentient beings on Earth, too.

The aim here is not to teach people how to be a perfect vegan, but rather to inspire the vast majority of people to do *something*. We all have the power to change the world, whether we silently choose our own food options, loudly attend climate rallies and protests, or enthusiastically write books and host podcasts to spread the word.

But who am I to write this book, anyway? Honestly, I'm just a regular person with a day job and a passion for this topic*. I'm not a climate scientist who gets paid to educate the public. I'm not a chef who has all day to concoct delicious vegan recipes. I'm not an athlete surrounded by coaches spending all my time dedicated to fitness and food. I don't even work in the vegan industry or have a vegan product to sell you. Just this book, actually. Mission accomplished—and thank you! But my mission goes much further than getting my thoughts—and copious amounts of research to back them up, mind you—down on paper.

I switched to vegan because it felt like the right thing to do for me and for my planet. Even though I'm not perfect at it, I still know I'm making a difference. I wrote this book because I feel called to talk about and share what I know, and hopefully to plant seeds that'll inspire others to make the switch. But,

---

* Shameless self-plug coming up: Actually, just before this book went to print, I delivered a TEDx talk on this topic, too.

mostly, I wanted to help those who were *struggling* with being vegan—because the struggle can be very real. I mean, let's face it—it's a whole new world. Many people have tried and then quit because it was just too hard to be perfect, and I wish I could have reassured them that they were on the right path and that whatever they could do was helpful. With this book, I know that I can share some things that worked for me—from tangible actions to mindset shifts—and I know that what I've learnt can help others.

Uncovering all the negative ways the animal industry impacts the world keeps me motivated to say no to animal products, and learning about the health benefits of a varied plant-based diet keeps me excited about what I'm adding to my plate instead of removing from it. But my transition to vegan wasn't straightforward and easy—in fact, it's still going (we'll talk more about transitions in Part 3). It's a big task to undertake and it can't be done overnight.

When I started this journey, I wanted to become clear on it myself. If I was going to change my whole life around by giving up the foods I've grown up with and learning to enjoy ingredients I used to think were weird, like tofu, I wanted to make sure it was true. So, I dug into the research. I started by reading books and watching documentaries, but then I looked up their references and read the reports and the studies directly. Something would spark a new question, and then I'd head down another rabbit hole. My research studies at university taught me critical thinking, and I learnt to differentiate science from marketing (and there's a *lot* of marketing.) One thing I'm really good at is absorbing a wide range of inputs, distilling the key ideas, and teaching them to others. And that's what you're getting with this book.

Introduction

In Part 1, I'll take you on a journey through my research to uncover what's so bad about the animal industry. Besides climate change and the exploitation of animals (and how it links to our own humanity), there's all the marketing and myths that keep the worst of it hidden, to make us believe that eating animals is normal, good for us, and done ethically.

Part 2 helps us let go of perfection. We may believe that what we eat is a personal choice, yet it's driven by many underlying social and psychological factors that influence our choices well before we get to the supermarket and decide what to have for dinner. We're humans who have to make choices in a complicated society, not to mention complicated internal minds, too. We'll explore how the 'perfect vegan' simply doesn't exist, and the psychology behind why perfection isn't the goal, anyway.

Finally, in Part 3, I'll leave you with specific actions you can take to support yourself on this journey. I've read plenty of books that get me all fired up but that leave me with an uneasy feeling of, 'Well, what the hell do I do now? Where do I go from here?' From simple food swaps to how to read scientific studies, you'll be equipped with the tools to make the decisions that are right for you.

At the end of the book, you'll find appendices with resources for more information, and, of course, a well-detailed reference list.

When you've reached the end of everything I'm about to share with you, you'll feel more confident in doing veganism the way that works for you, and you'll have the language to explain your reasons. You'll have learnt something that made you go, 'Huh—I never thought of it like that before.'

And you'll feel inspired and compelled to *do something*.

Part 1

What's So Wrong with the Animal Industry?

CHAPTER 1: Climate Change

I'm embarrassed to admit this now, but I used to think that saving the environment was simply so we could have pretty spaces to live in and look at and enjoy. You know, gorgeous trails to go hiking in, and lush green, sprawling parks for picnics and playgrounds in our cities. I thought that protecting the Amazon rainforest from deforestation was simply a matter of pride; after all, it's so big and had been around so long, like a national treasure that we should put in a museum to admire. I honestly believed that biodiversity was only good for keeping bird watchers entertained and for discovering interesting creatures in David Attenborough documentaries. Same goes for the whales—it would be sad if they were no longer around, but aside from whale-watching tourism going out of business, what was the big deal?

Cue even more embarrassment. Oh, how naïve I was! Since beginning this research, I've learnt how vital these intricate systems are to the delicate balance of life on Earth. The lesson on environment I remembered learning from primary school was that ecosystems worked in harmony, and that any small introduction or removal from an area could wreak havoc—like the 13 rabbits introduced for sport hunting in newly colonised Australia that within 50 years had become a plague across the entire continent—so of course I figured that adults in the world were protecting these precious environments. I didn't realise that not only were the majority of people unaware of what was happening, but that several industries were actually *wilfully* destroying whole ecosystems and introducing toxic, irreversible changes.

However, when there was a ban on travel, tourism, and public gatherings due to the COVID pandemic, we witnessed how quickly the earth can bounce back in some areas[1]. Like sparse coral reefs—untouched for only a few weeks—repopulating themselves with fish[2], and pollution being reduced in usually smog-filled cities as a result of all the cars being off the roads (like in northern India, where residents could finally see the Himalayas for the first time in a generation[3]). It just goes to show how resilient Mother Earth is, and you know what? I've come to realise that she doesn't need us. Nope. She'll be absolutely fine when humans aren't even a memory anymore. If we disappear now, it might take a few thousand years, but she'll eventually return to pre-industrial climate levels when we stop intervening. The Earth doesn't need us—*we need her*. If we humans want to continue calling this planet home and live comfortably on its surface, we need to do whatever we can to look after what our ancestors have for millennia called 'Mother'.

Chapter 1: Climate Change

Is It Global Warming or Cooling?

When I was in school, we learned about global warming. We all did, right? But there was always this contradictory crowd who insisted, 'No, it's global *cooling*', and it kind of made us all wonder what the real deal was. For many decades, the debate raged on about whether we're getting cooler or hotter, rather than trying to do anything about what was actually happening[4]. No wonder so many people turned a blind eye and a deaf ear. What we now refer to as 'climate change' is neither uniform cooling nor warming of the *weather*, but a warming of our planet's *atmosphere*, which results in extreme and unpredictable weather events that are experienced differently around the world. So when we see English airports being closed in the spring because of unseasonable snow[5], record heatwaves in arctic Moscow[6], and Australian floodwaters covering areas the size of France and Germany[7], these are all examples of how our climate is changing—all due to a seemingly tiny rise in global temperatures of 1° Celsius compared to the early Industrial baseline way back between 1880 and 1890.

We know this is a fact, because clever scientists have been able to model planetary temperatures going back thousands of years. And even though the models differ based on their instruments of measurement, they all clearly show a sharp increase in averages around the start of the 20th century[8]. In fact, it's been around 75 consecutive years since we've experienced even one year below the Industrial average temperature[9], and nine of the ten hottest years on record have occurred since 2013 (Figure 1).

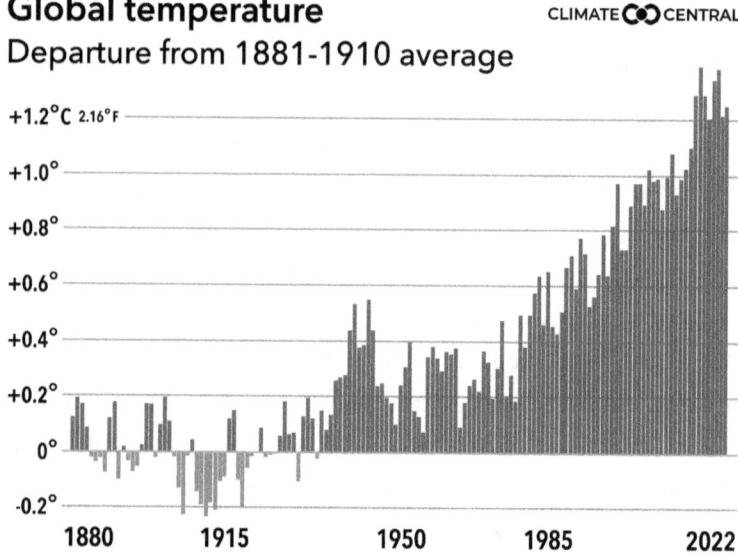

Figure 1. Global Temperature Increases

The scary thing about these models is that this trend is exponential. The warmer we get, the faster we *continue* to get warmer. It's a snowball effect (and that's just a metaphor, not a nod to the 'global cooling' crowd). Even if there's still some contention around whether global warming is manmade or natural—and there is*—we can all agree that it's happening and that its effects will be devastating.

Here's what we don't want: at 2 degrees, we'll see sea levels rise by several feet, remapping coastlines around the world and making popular coastal cities virtually uninhabitable; 99% of

---

* Is it politically incorrect to roll my eyes at this argument?

Chapter 1: Climate Change

coral reefs will die from sun bleaching; 25% of animal species and plants will face extinction; food yields will reduce due to droughts, floods, and heat waves; and global conflict will break out due to water shortages, food system collapse, and billions of climate migrants moving into occupied lands[10-14]. Even if by some Herculean effort we limit our warming to 1.5°—which many scientists are now saying is out of reach—we'll still see rising sea levels, floods, droughts and heatwaves, species extinctions, and a 90% loss of coral reefs[15].

Let's talk about coral reefs for a second. We can easily imagine how droughts and floods impact humans (from a basic reductionist standpoint, droughts mean our food doesn't grow, and floods mean we lose our homes and property), but I also wondered why we should be so concerned about the loss of coral reefs. Aren't they just good for stunning scenery as we're snorkelling? An Insta-worthy backdrop for that scuba selfie? I looked it up, and learned that without coral reefs, our shorelines have no protection. Therefore, our coastal cities would be battered by waves and erosion, causing human populations to retreat further inland to survive (in other words, climate migration). In addition, coral reefs make up only 1% of our ocean, yet are home to a *quarter* of all marine life. And no, that's not just important for tourism and divers—the small species who live there also produce around 50-80% of the ocean's oxygen[16,17]. Which kind of comes in handy when we humans want to, you know, breathe and such. There are many things in this world we can survive without—TV, trans fats, and parking tickets, for starters—but oxygen isn't one of them.

Scarily, this isn't some far away, 'not-in-my-lifetime' sci-fi scenario. Scientists are predicting the disruption to begin as early as 2030, and they've been talking about it for a long time[18]. Although we've had warnings since the 1950s, and the first Earth Day was in 1970, the global science community didn't begin to unite and agree until the 1980s. And, since an unfortunate trait of humanity is to ignore problems until they actually begin to affect us personally, it wasn't until the early 2000s that governments started to get on onboard.

In 2015, the Paris Agreement[19] was finally signed by 196 countries as a legally binding agreement to do everything we can to limit global warming to 2°C, with a target of keeping it under 1.5° by 2030. However, since we've already established that global warming isn't uniform across the world, some areas are already experiencing global average increases of *above* 1.5°, like Bangladesh with their extreme tropical cyclones and flooding[20], Africa with their devastating droughts[21], and Spain with their climate migrants from Africa who are escaping those droughts[22]. In 2020, the Intergovernmental Panel on Climate Change (IPCC) issued a stark warning that we have a remaining global CO_2 budget of around 460 gigatonnes for a 50% chance of keeping our planet under 1.5°[23]—and yet only three years later, we may have used half of that already[24].

Let's introduce why CO_2 is so important, and why we have a budget. Don't worry, I promise this book is an enjoyable read, not a complex academic thesis. So, without taking you through a degree in climate science, I'll summarise the key points. For a detailed explanation in plain language, I'll refer you to Jonathan Safran Foer's excellent book *We Are the Weather*[25], which is one of the best and clearest descriptions of the issue I've come across. But basically, carbon dioxide is one of many natural gases in our atmosphere that's essential for life. It helps to keep the heat of the sun inside the planet

Chapter 1: Climate Change

so that plants (read: food) will grow and so that we can live comfortably on the surface and not underground in caves. However, if there's too much CO_2 in the atmosphere, it traps too much heat, not only making things hot and uncomfortable, but increasing condensation which then turns into precipitation (rain) in the clouds. This happens in smaller, more concentrated areas, causing extreme rainfall in some places and extreme drought in others, which is what's causing all our unpredictable weather events in places we never expected.

Isn't It Natural?

Okay, but aren't we exaggerating a little bit? How can we tiny little humans be responsible for affecting something as powerful as Mother Nature? Surely all this chatter about 'too much CO_2 in the atmosphere' is just part of the planet's natural cycle, yes? A little ebb and flow, just like the glaciers of Ice Ages past? Ah, again with my naivety. If only it were that easy—or innocent.

Although our data and science *does* show the planet cycling through periods of cooling and heating, these happen over thousands—even millions—of years, not *this* fast. Data going back 800,000 years tracks many of these cycles, and includes several Ice Ages during this time. While we tend to hover between 200 to 250 parts per million of CO_2 in the atmosphere, you can clearly see that we've never had more than 300ppm until the past 200 years, which coincides with the start of the Industrial Revolution (Figure 2). Since the 1950s, when our intensive manufacturing and industrial farming ramped up, CO_2 has shot up to over 400ppm and continues to rise[26].

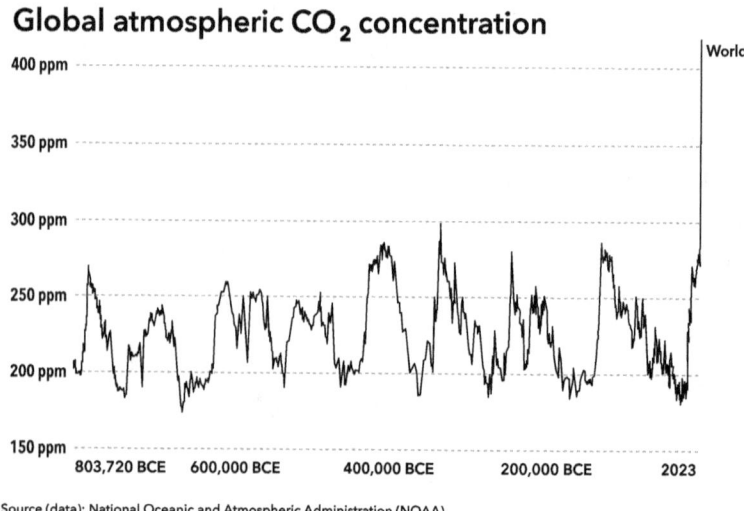

Figure 2: Global Atmospheric CO_2 Concentration Over 800,000 Years

Scientists say that humanity is in the midst of the sixth great extinction on this planet. Read that again. We're *in the midst* of it—it's not just some far-off prediction. It's easy to discount this kind of warning as nothing more than a sensationalistic doomsday prophesy or just something that makes a flashy headline, but the science speaks for itself. And currently, things are looking fairly ominous. The largest of these mass extinctions was 250 million years ago. Dubbed 'The Great Dying', it started when a volcano chain erupted, releasing massive amounts of CO_2 into the atmosphere. This blanket of CO_2 eventually raised global temperatures by ten degrees, which suffocated the oceans and killed off 96% of marine life and 70% of land life[27]. Today, our industrial

Chapter 1: Climate Change

processes are releasing CO_2 into the atmosphere *ten times faster* than those volcanoes. Read that again, too.

And where are we getting all this carbon from? Carbon was neatly tucked away by Mother Nature's ingenious solution of using it to build the roots and trunks of plants and trees, and inside the bodies of marine creatures as they sank to the bottom of the ocean floor. These natural storage facilities are now being very quickly dredged up, dug up, ripped out, and burnt down to their composite gases, which float serenely into the atmosphere where they get trapped and begin to wreak absolute havoc on our planet.

In addition to going all *Storage Wars* on Mother Nature, our human activities are adding even more emissions. Thanks to the media, you're likely aware of the fossil fuel industry and its contribution to this global catastrophe. You've also likely caught wind of celebrities being shamed for their high-emission private jets or, conversely, lauded for their all-electric luxury yachts. And since you picked up this book about veganism, you may also have heard about the impact of animal agriculture, although I doubt you would have seen *that* on the evening news. Mainstream headlines are more focused on Kim Kardashian's butt than the fact that she's vegan. And while that butt is lovely, I suppose, I doubt it will save the planet (though stranger things have been known to occur with that family).

Here's where we stand: in 2006, the United Nations Food and Agricultural Organization (UNFAO) released *Livestock's Long Shadow*[28], a report calling out the animal agriculture industry as being one of the top two or three contributors to global greenhouse gas (GHG) emissions. The energy sector is obviously the greatest contributor, but, depending on the source, animal agriculture is either more than or about the same as the entire transport industry (around 16%)—that's all the personal cars, public transport, international flights, and fleets of freight trucks combined[26]. These figures come from a combination of emissions within production and packaging, feed given to animals, methane from livestock, and land clearing, but they don't include grazing land for livestock.

Due to this omission, other researchers, notably World Watch Institute[29], actually suggest this percentage to be as high as 51%. Its report from 2009 points out that the UNFAO report undercounted, overlooked, and misreported several figures, even conflicting some of its own previous calculations. They say that the UNFAO report did not account for by-products and downstream effects of livestock such as the carbon sequestration potential of land in use; that it underestimated the warming effects of methane (it's 86 times more potent than CO_2 in a 20-year period); and that it even left out the fishing industry completely. Even with the UNFAO conservative calculations, whatever the exact figure, we can agree it's not a trifling amount.

The United Nations are the group of experts we've collectively nominated to represent our best interests. Way back in 2006, their *Livestock's Long Shadow* report advised all governments that animal agriculture should be a major consideration in upcoming climate policy, and then in 2010, they upped their recommendations and said that the majority of the world needs to shift to a plant-based diet in order to avoid climate catastrophe[30]. Has *your* government told you at any point in the past decade to switch to a plant-based

Chapter 1: Climate Change

diet? Not an investigative news report, not a documentary, and not an influencer—the *government*. Didn't think so. Why not? Even though the science is wildly clear, corporations and industry giants are protecting their profits, and governments are tied down by lobbyists. Even in Al Gore's ground-breaking documentary *An Inconvenient Truth*, there was no mention of agriculture's role. I'll cover more on these troubling thoughts in Chapter 3: Marketing & Myths.

So what can we do? The list of actions at the end of *An Inconvenient Truth* are kind of vague and almost laughable ('Speak up in your community! Run for congress! Pray!'). Somehow, I think it'll take more than a few Hail Marys or Om Shantis to halt our pending climate calamity. Chad Frischmann gave an enlightening TED Talk[31] with a list of 100 possible solutions, as proposed by *Project Drawdown*, a world-leading resource for global climate issues. However, much of them require big, systemic change, and they're more than an individual can tackle on their own (such as converting to clean energy).

Is Green Energy Any Better?

The jury is out on this one. 'Clean' energy mining sometimes generates more environmental damage and toxic waste than is currently required to mine fossil fuels. In her powerful TED Talk, Olivia Lazard[33] shares how electric vehicles require six times the inputs compared to standard vehicles. My hope is that this disparity will reverse itself as the technology becomes better, cheaper, and more effective, like how computers used to take up whole rooms and cost billions, and now we all have an affordable one right in our own pockets.

Switching to clean energy isn't as simple as changing your home energy supplier or buying a Tesla: oil and gas power the world. They're not just fuel for our cars—they also power the mining that digs up the rare earth materials to make the solar panels and electric car batteries for our green energy machines. It's certainly possible to move away from fossil fuels—it's just not a quick fix, and it's rarely an individual action. Even if the whole world completely eliminated the fossil fuel industry and switched to clean nuclear fusion—and we're not sure if that's even possible within ten years—we're still going to blow over our global carbon budget if we keep eating meat and dairy.

To help clarify the actions an individual can take, a team of environmental scientists published a report in 2017[32] to highlight the four most impactful individual actions:

- ✓ Have fewer children
- ✓ Fly less
- ✓ Consider giving up your personal car
- ✓ Switch to a plant-based diet

Out of these top four recommendations, only a plant-based diet is something that we can do immediately and without much effort, and at least three times a day from now on. How often do you decide whether or not to have a baby? And you certainly can't put them back once you've got them (though it may be tempting once they enter the 'terrible twos').

This report shows that if we eat meat and take just one international flight per year, we've already used up our personal carbon budget based on our projections to remain below the 2° temperature rise. In a typical Western diet, food choices contribute to around 10-30% of our personal emissions[34], and switching to a plant-based diet can halve that amount[35]. Yes, it requires effort to change what's on your plate, but not as much effort as trying to manoeuvre your IKEA flatpacks on the bus or walking to the supermarket and only buying what you can carry after having given up your personal car.

So, while shifting our diets away from animal agriculture will not be our sole saviour in climate change, there's no solution without it. And GHGs are only part of the climate puzzle—animal agriculture is also the leading cause of other global catastrophes that upset the delicate balance of life on earth: deforestation, ocean dead zones, freshwater use, and water pollution, as well as ocean plastic and biodiversity loss.

Looking at the whole industry from a top-down and Earth-centred approach, animal agriculture is an incredibly inefficient way to feed humans. The rest of this chapter will explore the disproportionate amounts of land, freshwater, and feed that go into producing a very small percentage of calories and protein for human consumption, along with the large percentage of negative consequences already mentioned. Individual companies don't even pay for these consequences, but every individual on the planet does—and with much more than their bank accounts.

No Company Would Be Run Like This

Let's address the massive inefficiency of our global meat industry. I think we'd all agree that if the Earth was a business, the CEO would be fired for mismanagement. A huge number of resources are used to produce a *lower* output than what went in. And not only is the input/output of resources unbalanced, we're also stripping these resources faster than the Earth can replace them. These individual corporations in the animal industry are like the middle managers of a business, climbing the corporate ladder with their own goals and budgets, without care for how the company as a whole performs as long as their own team is getting ahead. Each manager looks like they're winning because their team's balance sheet shows profit, but no one is measuring the waste on the way in or the damage on the way out. And they all have so much money that they can effectively bribe the CEO to turn a blind eye.

The thing is, this isn't a business that's going to go bust, after which we'll all sigh and say we saw it coming and that the CEO should be punished—this is our *planet*. If it goes belly up, no one will be around to deal with the fallout. You might think that humanity is too big to fail, but unlike when the banks failed in 2008, there won't be anyone to bail us out. Who would come? Where would we go? There's no galactic Mum and Dad whose couch we can crash on for a few months while we turn our lives around. This is *it*. We need to step up and begin adulting. Unfortunately, we're all in this 'Company Earth' together, so it's no good looking outward and saying, 'They're bad.' If they go down, we all go down, so we all need to *do something*, and we need to do it now.

Phew. Have I got you all hot and bothered? In my defence, it likely wasn't me, actually—it was more likely the rising global temperatures, or maybe even some en-masse cow flatulence. In any event, something definitely stinks here, so whatever's got you all riled up (because, by this point, I'd hope that you would be), let's look at some stats on this.

Chapter 1: Climate Change

Land and Water Use

Not all land is suitable for farming. Of the actual land on Earth (not ocean), only about 70% of it is habitable—the rest is barren desert or glaciers. And this will likely come as a huge shock to you (I know that I was certainly blown away): *only 1% of land is urban development*—that's all the bustling cities, gridlocked roads, towering skyscrapers, colossal pyramids, and (for better or for worse) addictive fast-food joints that humanity has constructed. Of the habitable land, we use nearly half for agriculture; the rest is forest and scrub. Now here's where the inefficiency comes in: of the half of all arable land that agriculture uses, *animal* agriculture takes up more than 80% of that, yet it provides only 18% of the total calories in the world[36]. We get the remaining 82% of our calories from plants, which only need 16% of farming land. Check out Figure 3 below. If we ate 100% of our calories from plants, we'd only need about 25% of available land[37]. This is important, because our population is going to have two billion more people within a couple of decades. Two. *Billion*. More. Within 20 years or so. And there's no more space to add more farms, unless we tear down forests or figure out how to grow food on glaciers.

Let's look a little closer at the agricultural land used for livestock, as the total of 82% includes crops used as livestock feed. The inefficiency here is that when we feed animals, they use most of that energy just to stay alive, and we get a much smaller percentage at the other end when the animal itself is converted to food. We lose at least 75% of calories this way, and the conversion ratio of beef is not even 2% (see Figure 4)[37]. It just doesn't make logical sense, does it?

Total global land use for food production

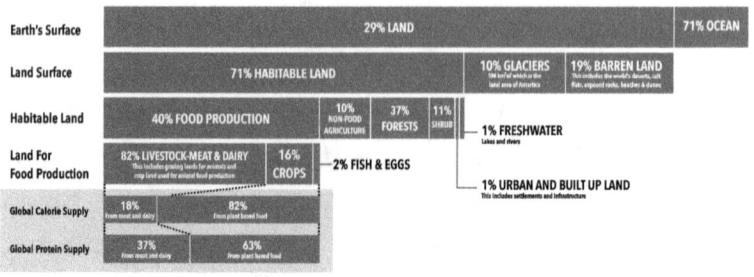

Source: Adapted from WWF (2020) Bending the Curve

Figure 3: Global Split of How We Use Our Land*

Percentage of calories from feed retained in final product (energy efficiency)

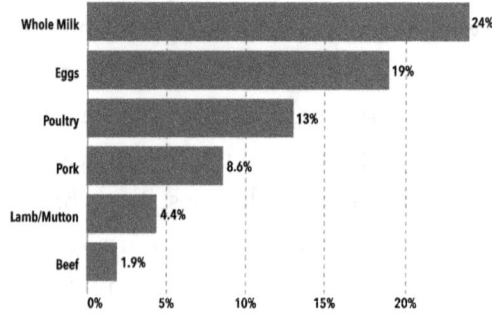

Source (data): Alexander el at (2016). Human appropriation of land for food: The role of diet. Global environmental change
Source (graph): OurWorldinData.org

Figure 4: Feed Conversation Ratio for Various Animal Products

---

* When I first wrote this section, the land-use data came from *Our World in Data*[38], but the WWF report is more up to date, and it unfortunately shows an increasing trend in the amount of arable land being used for animal agriculture, up to 82% from 77%.

Chapter 1: Climate Change

This inefficiency is further demonstrated in a report using USDA data itself, reviewing annual productivity of the land by food product[39]. It compared meat products to plant products and found that cows generate 150 pounds of beef per acre, whereas fruits and vegetables generate 17,000 pounds per acre. Let me just pause there to recap: 150 pounds to *17,000 pounds*. Yes, we need to eat more veggies to get the same number of calories as from beef, but only about four times as much, not 113 times. That little acre could feed you for about three months if you ate nothing but beef (ew, can you imagine the meat sweats?!), or for nearly *four years* if you ate the 17,000 pounds of veggies (Figure 5). And you'd get a varied diet, too.

That calculation is based on *calories*, and if we were to compare based on *protein* content, we'd need only about twice as many grains compared to beef. That means 300 pounds of grains to equal the protein content in 150 pounds of beef from this one acre. And since grains produce about 6,000 pounds per acre, we'd only need 5% of that acre to achieve the same protein density as the beef from a full acre (Figure 6).

Yearly production output per acre of beef versus vegetables (calories)

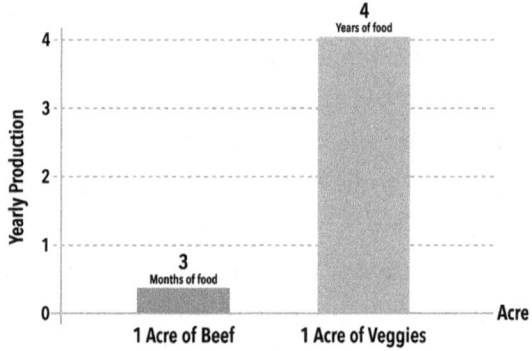

Figure 5: One Acre of Cow Versus One Acre of Vegetables

Land required to achieve comparative protein output of beef versus wholegrains

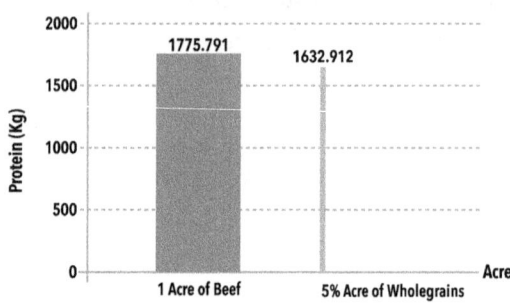

Figure 6: One Acre of Cow Produces Approximately the Same Protein as 5% of an Acre of Grains.

Chapter 1: Climate Change

Looking back to Figure 3, we also see that although animals take up more than 80% of our land, they only provide around a third of our global protein. When we break down land use by individual food item, it's obvious to see why. A cursory glance at Figure 7 shows how disproportionate the land use is, with lamb and beef needing 20 to 30 times more land than common plant-based protein sources like beans and grains.

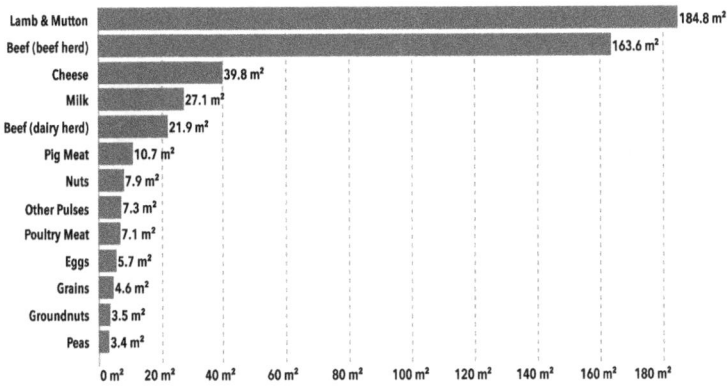

Source (data): Joseph Poore and Thomas Nemecek (2018). Additional calculation by our World in Data
Source (graph): OurWorldinData.org

Figure 7: Land Use per 100g of Protein[40],

It's pretty clear, right? Without even doing the math, we could feed significantly more people on plants than animal meat.

~

Water use tells more of the same story. Agriculture uses more than two-thirds of our global freshwater supplies every year, and the majority of that is for livestock. As it stands, only 0.5% of all the water on earth is accessible freshwater available for us to drink[41], and 20% of that goes to the animals we eat instead[42]. Crazily enough, only about 2% is what they drink themselves—and 98% is used for growing the grains and pastures they feed on[43]. This doesn't only apply to feedlot cows that are fed imported grains grown on someone else's farm; while pasture-raised cows are happily munching away on grassy, green fields, industrial-sized sprinklers are watering the other four fields they rotate on throughout the year.

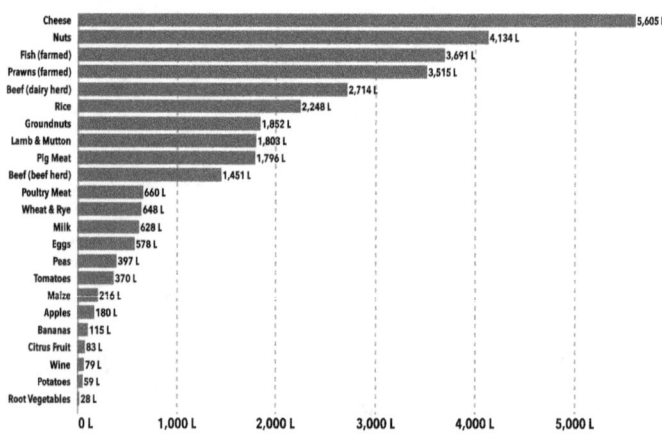

Source (data): Joseph Poore and Thomas Nemecek (2018)
Source (graph): OurWorldinData.org

Figure 8. Water Requirements for Food Type Based on Weight

When we break it down by food type, we can clearly see how much water goes into each kind of product. Whether

Chapter 1: Climate Change

we're measuring by calories, protein, or kilograms, animal products need much more water than plants. The water requirement for beef is eight to nine times as much as for the same calories of veggies and grains[44]. For 100 grams of protein, cheese requires triple the water use of beef, and beef needs triple again compared to lentils and beans[45]. Have a look at Figure 8 above to see the difference in water use per kilogram of final product. This is why a cheeseburger is equivalent to around 660 gallons (2,500 litres) of water, or, leaving the kitchen sink running for five and a half hours. Imagine leaving the tap running while you went to the shops, bought ingredients for dinner, cooked dinner, washed the dishes, watched an episode of *MasterChef*, and played with your kids in the new living room paddling pool. Rethinking that run to the drive-thru yet?

Even though some plant products need more water and land than others, plenty of studies have evaluated different types of diets, and they all agree that a plant-based diet is better overall for the health of the planet. *Our World in Data* shows how a vegan diet needs only a quarter of the current cropland in use[37]. One systematic review analysed diet studies ranging from seven days to 27 years, and found that the vegan diet had the lowest emissions and water use, making it the most sustainable choice in terms of environmental footprint[46]. A 2020 report by WWF, *The Restorative Power of Planet-Based Diets*[36], echoes this. Figure 9 below clearly shows the global impact of various diets, with vegan being the least-emitting, and standard Western the highest. This report also explains how the majority of biodiversity loss and GHG emissions come from land use, with a typical Western diet needing three billion hectares of grassland, while a plant-exclusive diet requires zero. *Zero.* If we were able to restore only a third of that grassland to forest, we'd not only increase our biodiversity, but we'd be able to sequester 205 gigatonnes of carbon—which is two-thirds of all carbon released since the industrial era, and nearly half of our total remaining carbon budget.

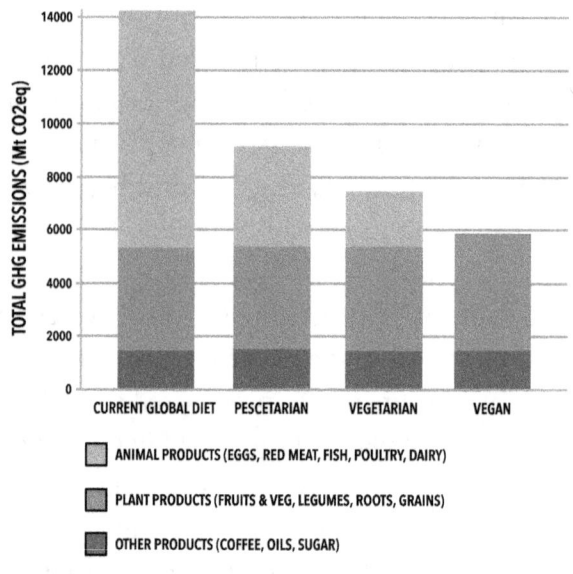

Source: Adapted from WWF (2020) Bending the Curve

Figure 9: Global Emissions Based on Diet Type (Source: WWF)

One of the most often-cited studies is Poore and Nemecek's landmark paper, *Reducing Food's Environmental Impacts Through Producers and Consumers*[47]. In this meta-analysis,*

---

* What's a meta-analysis? What's a systematic review? Don't worry, we'll cover this in Part 3 when we learn about evaluating evidence. (Hint: they're really good quality sources.)

Chapter 1: Climate Change

they compiled data from more than 38,000 farms across 119 countries to calculate the environmental impact of 40 types of foods. They evaluated land use, freshwater withdrawals, and emissions across the full lifecycle from production inputs (such as feed, fertilizer choice, and soil condition) to consumption (including packaging and transport). Their findings show that a plant-exclusive diet reduces emissions by 70% compared to a standard Western diet. Even the lowest-impact animal foods still carried a greater environmental burden than the highest-impact vegetable foods.

This means that if the world switched to a plant-based diet, we'd halve our emissions and free up around two-thirds of land for rewilding, even with our growing population. We'd create forests, wildlife, natural carbon sinks, and biodiversity to increase the strength of our ecosystem. And we could also save 61 trillion gallons of drinking water**.

Food Waste

Our choice of diet also has a disproportionate effect on emissions in food waste. Half of all food waste happens at the consumer level, but not all of it has the same environmental impact. Plant foods make up nearly half of all waste by weight, yet only contribute 12% of emissions. Animal products make up only a third of waste by weight, but account for 73% of emissions[73].

** Calculations based on Heinke and colleagues' (2020) report on global water use in livestock production[48], which shows that animal agriculture uses 4,387km3 of water for animal feed, 94% of which is green water. Therefore, 6% of agriculture use is blue (drinking) water. Six percent equals 263km3 which is 61 trillion gallons/230 trillion litres.

~

By 2050, we're expected to have ten billion people on the planet, all while experiencing severe droughts, heatwaves, floods, and food shortages. We're supposed to feed *more* people under *harsher* conditions, and we need to use less land than we currently do. Due to dwindling freshwater reservoirs, scientists are saying that by 2050, we'll need to be on a global plant-based diet to avoid climate wars. However, the World Health Organisation is warning us that by 2025, half of the world will already be experiencing water shortages[49,50].

Feeding animals to humans just does not make mathematical sense when you consider that we can use less land to grow fewer crops and use less water to feed us the same amount of calories and protein. We'd save around 75% of currently used arable land and still have enough to feed a population of ten billion, with the added benefit of rewilding the remaining land to speed up our drawdown of excess carbon from the atmosphere. You can see why big names like the UN, IPCC, and Arnold Schwarzenegger recommend a global shift to a plant-based diet. And when the Terminator tells you to do something, you do it (or you at least *strongly* consider it).

And yet, because these middle managers of Company Earth—our animal agriculture corporations—don't seem to own calculators, they're pushing for more and more space to continue the current system, which is what's driving deforestation as they clear land to grow crops or put animals to pasture. And it's at an astounding speed. Every year, we lose an area approximately the size of Panama[51]. This may help to put that thought into perspective: there are only 88

Chapter 1: Climate Change

'Panamas' in the Amazon.* Importantly, though, it's not just an Amazonian or Indonesian thing—animal agriculture even drives 79% of the deforestation in Australia[52].

Why is this scary? As mentioned earlier, I used to think we were just protecting the rainforest because of the colourful parrots and cheeky monkeys who live there, and because it's a nice thing to do. But actually, it's *essential* for human life. Forests are the literal lungs of the planet. Through the process of photosynthesis, they capture CO_2 from the atmosphere and break it down into oxygen, which is released for us to breathe, and into carbon, which is used to build their trunks and roots, storing it for many hundreds of years until they decompose naturally and continue the cycle of life. Mother Nature sure knows what she's doing.

There's a two-fold impact of cutting down trees. First of all, when they're burnt (which most of the deforested land is), their stored carbon—sometimes hundreds of years of it—is released immediately into the atmosphere, speeding up the warming. Secondly, since trees would have continued to grow, there's no longer the ability to capture future carbon in this spot. So not only are we adding more greenhouse gas emissions, we're blocking any more from being sequestered. In 2021, scientists identified that the Amazon is now releasing more carbon than it captures, speeding up atmospheric warming[53]. Deforestation is like clearing space in our lungs to grow an extra stomach. It's trying to feed us while destroying the very thing that's keeping us alive.

---

* By land size. The 6.7 million square kilometres of the Amazon could hold 88 of the 75-square kilometre 'Panamas'.

You might've heard that deforestation is caused by the need for things like palm oil and soy, and you'd be right. However, palm oil is responsible for only about 7% of deforestation globally, whereas cattle ranching accounts for 40% (63% in the Amazon)[54]. Okay, so what about soy? Yes, soy is also responsible for 7% of deforestation (double that in the Amazon). Guess who eats soy? Yep, humans. But while we do eat tofu, edamame beans, and soy sauce, that only accounts for 7% of all soy grown globally, which usually comes from sustainable, non-GMO systems in Europe.

So where does the rest of it go? Oh, that's right, it's fed to livestock. Macho meat eaters thought they were avoiding soy, but nearly 80% of soy grown around the world is fed to animals destined for human consumption*[55]. Want to hear something extra inefficient about that? If humans ate the same number of calories from crops as they'd get from the animal that ate the crops, we'd only need to grow about a quarter of them[38].

Yep, we're destroying the lungs of our planet to feed the animals we eat who provide us with only a quarter of the calories we feed them in the first place. And it's weird, because it isn't even a big secret: the animal agriculture corporations closely measure their 'feed conversion ratio' to try and get it as low as possible, although they do this from a cost-saving perspective, not a 'we-need-a-planet-to-live-on' one.

And the inefficiency of animal feed doesn't stop there. Remember, we use 20% of our drinking water for animal agriculture, and it's not because cows are thirsty. The reason

---

* The remaining 13% is for oil and biofuels.

Chapter 1: Climate Change

is worthy of repeating: it's because we use that water to grow the crops to feed the animals that only provide us with a quarter of the calories we could've got from eating their food instead. And before you think, 'But I don't want to eat that much soy!', you don't have to. We can grow other crops on that land, too. And, actually, it's better for the health of our soils if we grow a variety of rotated crops. Switching things up keeps the soil fertile and full of the essential nutrients that end up in our food.

It's in Our Oceans, Too

They say that we learn something new every day, so here's a doozy for you: deforestation doesn't just happen on land—it happens in the oceans as well. How can this be? Are bulldozers charging through coral reefs? Not exactly, although it's not far off the truth. But first let's explore why oceans are crucial to life on earth.

If the forest is our lungs, the ocean is our breath. The National Oceanic and Atmospheric Administration (NOAA) says that between 50-80% of the oxygen we breathe comes from our oceans[56], and our oceans store around a third of the planet's carbon[57]. It all starts with tiny microplankton. They use photosynthesis to capture CO_2, releasing oxygen for us and storing carbon for themselves, just like trees on land. When microplankton are eaten by fish, the carbon bioaccumulates (it sticks around in their bodies). Those fish are then eaten by larger fish, and so on and so on, and when those large fish die naturally, they sink to the bottom of the ocean, taking their accumulated carbon with them. Incidentally, poo from whales, the largest of our sea creatures, also contains high concentrates of iron and nitrogen, both vital nutrients that encourage the growth of microplankton, reinforcing the cycle and further enhancing the ocean's ability to store carbon. Again, Mother Nature's got it all figured out: she's clearly thought this through—whale poo and all.

The ocean is home to a rich store of sequestered carbon and a diverse array of life. She supports all life on this planet: without her, we literally wouldn't be able to breathe. However, the meat and fishing industries are destroying this wondrous ecosystem in the following ways:

Bottom trawling

Massive fishing trawlers are indiscriminately tearing up the forests of the ocean floor, destroying marine ecosystems and habitats, and also releasing carbon 20 times faster than burning the Amazon[58,59].

Bycatch

Both trawling and long-line fishing are responsible for species loss, extinction risk, and removing carbon through the unnecessary deaths of billions of aquatic lives per year. Globally, every time a mountain of sea life is hauled onto the fishing vessel, 40% of that is bycatch. Besides turtles, dolphins, sharks, and seahorses, even the fish that we'd otherwise eat can be considered 'bycatch' if they're not what that particular trawler needed to fill their quota on that particular outing[60].

Pollution

Toxic run-off from farms, mostly pesticides and nitrogen from manure pools, is reaching our oceans and causing algae blooms[61]. This not only pollutes our domestic rivers along the way, but it causes eutrophication—massive algae overgrowth that sucks oxygen out of the water and suffocates fish (otherwise known as dead zones).

Plastics

Between 50-70% of the plastic in the ocean is from discarded commercial fishing gear[62,63]. Besides the issue of 'ghost fishing' that traps many dolphins, whales, and turtles, nets break down into microplastics, and then small fish eat them. These microplastics can't be excreted as poo, so when they're eaten by larger fish, it bioaccumulates in their bodies, all the way up to the fish we eat. And yes, you're right: then it sticks around in *our* bodies and damages our health in a myriad of ways.

Eating farmed fish is unfortunately not a better solution, although I'd originally thought it was. For starters (and this was surprising to me), since most fish are carnivores who need to eat other fish, our fishing industries go out to sea in their big trawlers and cause all that environmental damage and then feed 20% of their catch to farmed fish[64]. Yes, you read that right: farmed fish are fed wild-caught fish. Why don't we just eat the wild-caught fish? The feed-conversion ratio plays out here, too: one study found that Scottish salmon, for example, produced 179,000 tonnes of farmed salmon for consumption, yet over that same time, 460,000 tonnes of wild-caught fish had been fed to that salmon. And here's the kicker—about 90% of that wild-caught fish was, in fact, of higher nutrient quality than the final output of farmed salmon it was fed to[65]. Doesn't it blow your mind how stupid that is?

Farmed fish, due to their close-confinement conditions, are also hotbeds of lice and disease. Estimates say that 15-20%

are lost before they get to market[66], and all fish are treated with a cocktail of poisons to try and contain lice outbreaks—most of which end up in the fish flesh we consume. Due to the pesticides, chemicals, and antibiotics sprayed indiscriminately on farmed fish (even those which are caged in ocean pens), these toxins leak out into the surrounding seas affecting wild species, and the residue forms a thick sludge under the bottom of the nets. This sludge then ferments and releases methane into the atmosphere, with some reports showing that this is more than beef's methane contribution[67,68]. And there we were, pegging the poor cows as solely to blame for the methane problem. Sorry, divine bovine—we now realise that you're not entirely at fault.

One of the best things you can do for the environment is to not eat fish, but don't worry: you won't be missing any vital nutrients like omega-3s. We'll explore that further in an upcoming chapter.

Loss of Biodiversity

Again, and this demonstrates my ignorance before I looked into things properly, the value of biodiversity isn't just so that we can learn about tiny flying monkeys in Madagascar ('so cute!') or fish that create their own light hundreds of meters down in the sea ('how cool!'). Nature has created a delicate balance of ecosystems that support each other and rely on the interconnectedness of all life. The destruction of oceans and the deforestation of our lands (both driven by our demand for animal products) are the leading factors in biodiversity loss and the potential extinction of millions of species.

Knocking out even one species can lead to another

Chapter 1: Climate Change

being overrun, leading to the loss of their food source from overconsumption. Losing *their* food source means that *they'll* die out too, so whoever relies on them for food will either starve or adapt. And if they adapt to eating another food source, they'll be in competition for whoever already eats that food. Vicious cycle in action.

You can see how the whole system will unravel, and the damage isn't contained within the animal kingdom. Animals and plants are interconnected, so there's the risk that an overpopulation of some species will impact our own food production. Think swarms of locusts eating our crops, or no bees around to pollinate them. Mother Nature has spent millions of years bringing these systems into a delicate balance, with changes occurring minutely and over millennia. The way our current food production is ripping up and stripping the earth of her resources is threatening this system, and therefore our own way of life.

The current rate of biodiversity loss is unprecedented in human history, leading scientists to declare that we're in the midst of the sixth great extinction. In the last few centuries, over 1,000 species of plants and land animals have become extinct, with one million more under threat[69,70]. We've also depleted 90% of the world's fisheries since just the 1950s[71].

When forests are cut down, birds, ground mammals, insects, and many other types of living beings lose their homes and their food supply, and they can't always move to the forest next door—remember how every little space is its own perfect ecosystem? They often just die. Even the microbes and bacteria that live in the soil and give it its richness and diverse nutrients are being wiped out through monocropping, leading to poorer yields, less nutrients in our soils, and less ability to grow what we want, when we want.

A (bio)diverse environment is one that's resilient to drought, floods, pests, and all the other problems that are exacerbated by climate change. Animal agriculture is not only speeding up climate change through emissions—it's also the leading driver of this biodiversity loss and damage to systems that would otherwise have been protective. Worse still, it tries to hide it through denial, lobbying, misreporting, and misdirection. We'll explore this in a later chapter when we shed some light on their contributions to the Climate Change Counter Movement (CCCM)[72].

~

Regardless of the spin they try to put on it, the evidence is clear: the animal agriculture industry is damaging the environment through deforesting our lands and ocean floors, polluting our waterways, bellowing potent methane into our skies, and using more of Earth's valuable resources than it's providing back to us. This inefficient system would be dismantled and the CEO fired if it was run like a business. But the Earth is *not* a business: it's the home of every single person you know, every *thing* you've ever known, and every generation yet to come. Animal agriculture is doing this to make individual profits, without looking at the impact of the whole world, but it'll stop breeding animals if there's no market to buy them.

We need to come together and solve this problem. No individual, no single country, and not even one large billion-dollar corporation can do it alone. And we can't rely solely on loud, passionate vegans working tirelessly in advocacy groups to accomplish this—we *all* need to play our part. This is a test of our humanity, and whether we can overcome our desire for short-term pleasure and convenience to achieve long-term and sustainable benefit. As we'll see in Part 2 (and as you've likely gathered), that's easier said than done. But I absolutely know that it's possible.

However, even if there was a sustainable way to produce animals for food (which is a myth that we'll challenge soon), our humanity is still at risk due to the suffering that's inherent in the industry. Eating animals on the scale we do necessarily relies on the exploitation of one species by another, which we'll tackle in the next chapter. Treating our planet with respect and care also means that we need to honour the other sentient beings we share this home with. We're not the only beings on this planet—and we might not be here for long if we don't act now.

CHAPTER 2: Exploitation

At this point, we've learnt about how the animal industry is pillaging our natural environment and risking the habitability of our home. Now we turn to something we all know on some level, and yet we remain oblivious to its full extent: animal exploitation.

For me, climate change is the most urgent reason to be vegan, but most people do come into veganism for their love of animals, and this wouldn't be a book about vegans without addressing exploitation. It's obvious that animals have to die in order for us to eat them, but it's not just the killing that's the problem with this industry—it's the unnecessary torture, pain, and suffering along the way, not to mention the fact that it tries to hide the reality, pretend it's not that bad, and convince us that we need it. While my aim is to avoid sensationalism—no need for it, as the truth is bad enough!—I'm also not going to gloss over the horrors, and, just to arm you

Chapter 2: Exploitation

with a disclaimer, some of the facts I'll be covering may be discomforting to hear about.

The intention of this chapter is not to be an exhaustive study of everything that goes on. I simply want to highlight some of the terrible things you might not already know about. I'll share the common practices that shocked and saddened me to learn about, and the things that keep me grossed out enough to avoid animal products even when the environmental damage is less front-of-mind. The thought exercises I introduce will, hopefully, reveal the connection between what we do to animals and the risk to our own humanity. For wider coverage on this topic, there are plenty of well-researched works that I encourage you to explore, and I'll provide these in the resource list at the end of the book.

Note: I say 'what *we* do' not to imply that each of us individually commits these atrocities, but we certainly do as a collective society. As a greater whole, we're all still complicit in these actions whether we see them or not, because consuming and purchasing these products tells the industry that there's a demand for them.

Paul McCartney is quoted as saying, 'If slaughterhouses had glass walls, everyone would be vegetarian,' but we don't need glass walls to instinctively know what happens inside. We choose to remain oblivious for one reason: we really don't want to know. Social psychologist and educator Melanie Joy says, 'In close to three decades of speaking and teaching about animal agriculture, I have yet to see a person who doesn't cringe when witnessing how animals are turned into food.'

When I asked my family to watch *Cowspiracy*[1] so that they could understand my reasons for being vegan, my sister told me she won't watch it because she's 'not ready to know yet.' And you know what? I don't blame her, because I said exactly the same thing to my friend about a decade ago when she asked *me* to watch it.

We don't want to see it, because if we do, we'll have to accept it. And if we accept it, we know we would need to *do* something. And doing something about this issue literally means changing our whole lives around. It's far easier to continue pretending that we can't see what's going on inside. From conducting this research and speaking firsthand to slaughterhouse workers, I can tell you that the reality of what's inside—the common legal practices even in 'high-welfare' countries—is much worse than I allowed myself to imagine.

~

As I confessed at the start, I'm not much of an animal lover. (And if you've forgiven me for that, you obviously haven't tossed this book into the bin, so thank you.) Again, I'm glad animals exist, and I wish them no harm, but I just don't particularly have a desire to interact with them. I don't mind looking at them from afar, and I do love cute little doggies who don't shed hair and drool all over me (or yap too much). But regardless of my lack of gushing towards animals, it's clear to see that what we do to them, purely for pleasure or taste or convenience and simply because we *can*, is just not right.

Animals are mistreated and abused for the sake of inflated demand driven by profit-seeking corporations, when in our

Chapter 2: Exploitation

affluent Western society, we don't even *need* to get our nutrients from animals. If we wouldn't do this to a human, or even a cute little dog (even the loud, hairy ones), why would we do it to a cow or a pig or a chicken?

There are laws in place to prevent cruelty to pets, children, and our fellow humans. (Huh. That kind of sounded like I don't consider children to be human, didn't it? Trust me, I absolutely do, even though spending time with my three-year-old nephew sometimes makes me wonder.) But those laws go out the window on farms. Animal welfare laws have this loophole called 'customary farming exemptions', which basically means that if I had a pet cow, I couldn't brand it, cut its tail, or castrate it without anaesthesia, but it would be fine if it wasn't a pet and I was rearing it to be sold for someone to eat[2-4]. I wouldn't be allowed to pick up my pet cat by its tail, but it's fine to pick up farmed chickens by their wings. There are laws against leaving dogs in hot cars, but pigs can be transported several days across the desert in hot, cramped trucks with no food or water and without breaks. If it's a common practice in farming, it's exempt from animal welfare laws. So much for 'animal welfare'.

These double standards are pervasive and right under our noses. We all know it's not acceptable to chain up a dog in a small crate and starve him by feeding him nothing but liquid broth, so why is it legal to do exactly that with baby male calves in veal crates? What makes bestiality illegal, when on farms it's acceptable to insert an electronic prod into the anus of a pig[5], or a farmer's arm inside a cow's vagina? (Warning: You don't even want to know what they do to artificially inseminate a sheep, and I'd advise you not to google it.)

The Imperfect Vegan

Why do Westerners happily eat steak while virulently protesting the dog meat trade in countries where it's considered normal, even though other parts of the world are appalled that we eat steak? In Florida, how can a man be sentenced to one year in jail with three years' probation and a mental health evaluation for running over a row of ducklings with his lawnmower[6], yet every day in the same state tens of thousands of day-old chicks are minced in industrial macerators or just dumped into the bin, simply because males won't lay eggs[7]? We don't even know the real numbers of lives lost in this way because 'waste products' of the animal industry aren't counted.

The stark, dark truth is that animals in this industry aren't seen as sentient individuals. They are seen—and treated—as products, nothing more. They're counted in units of measurement, such as 'heads' of cattle, or referred to by their use, as in 'layer hens' or 'broiler chickens'. Fish aren't even counted individually, but by tonnage.

Animals are a commodity: resources that are ordered in the tens of thousands from a hatchery, or forcibly birthed in deplorable conditions and then weaned from their mothers too early, with the sole intention of growing them to slaughter weight as fast and as cheaply as possible. In most places, they're kept alive just long enough to be 'harvested', which is in childhood or adolescence for the majority—a fraction of their natural lives[8].

There is no individual care, and sick or injured animals are usually left to their own demise. Death before slaughter is an 'unfortunate' reality, and an acceptable percentage is accounted for in calculations and pricing. In chicken barns, for instance, it's a daily task for workers to walk the floor and

Chapter 2: Exploitation

pick out any dead birds, and in piggeries, any sickly piglets are 'thumped' (this is the official industry term, and I'll let you use your imagination) to death, often right in front of their mothers[9-12].

Traditional farming—referred to as 'animal husbandry' (which sounds a bit seedier than it actually is)—used to be about farmers working the land personally, knowing each of their animals individually, and allowing them to live their lives as free as possible on what the land could provide. While I've personally seen that some of this still exists, it's a tiny percentage: today, husbandry has been replaced by science. Huge, sterile, polluting factory farms have taken over the industry (and most of the original traditional farms), using technology and genetic engineering created by 'animal science' graduates from the big city, with no care for animal welfare beyond the bare minimum of survival relative to productivity and the basic standards required by law.

While it would be nicer for the animals to be reared outdoors where they have space to move, interact with each other socially, and exhibit natural instinctual behaviours like pecking and roosting, they're cheaper to raise and easier to control when brought inside the giant barns and feedlots. Globally, nearly three quarters of all animal food products now come from factory farms[13], with these factories supplying 99% of meat in the US[14]; 95% in Australia[15]; 73% in the UK[16]; and over 72% in Europe[17]. These figures only account for land animals, not the billions of farmed fish kept in captivity as well. These behemoth corporations have been swallowing up smaller traditional farmers, because they can't compete on price. Even though marketing would have us believe otherwise (as we'll explore in the next chapter), our traditional farming values have been lost.

In reality, welfare is inconvenient for the animal industry. The more it costs to look after an animal, the less profit the company makes. The faster an abattoir line moves, the more animals can be processed in a day[18]. Animals are supposed to be stunned before they're bled out, and bled out before they're skinned or boiled, but due to the speed of the lines, slaughterhouse workers admit that not a day goes by without animals making it past all those measures and still being alive when they get to the cutting room[19]. 'Nothing stops the line' as they say. It seems, in the animal industry at least, that nothing's more inefficient than care and empathy.

We're told that tail-docking and debeaking are done for the animals' welfare, but, in reality, it's done to protect the farmer's other units of production. The reason that farmed animals bite each other's tails, peck each other's infected sores, and turn to cannibalism is a well-documented response to the psychological trauma from their confinement and conditions[20,21].

And in fact, the same thing would happen to humans if we were kept in these conditions[22]. Since I don't feel a natural affinity with animals (am I forgiven yet?), the way I relate to this treatment is to imagine if it were done to humans.

Imagine that an alien species came to this planet and decided that we were good food. They obviously wouldn't hunt us to extinction (surely if they've figured out space travel, they're more intelligent than that), so they'd instead round us up and keep us in pens, and then figure out how to replicate us so that we can continue to supply their ravenous needs.

Chapter 2: Exploitation

Some of us would be sent to work, others sent to zoos or the science lab, but most of us would end up in cramped, dirty, disease-ridden confinement in an endless cycle of breeding and having our children eaten. Our only revenge would be the new zoonotic diseases[23] we develop because of our conditions that hopefully would jump the human-alien barrier and infect our captors, like SARS, swine-flu, or COVID-19.

If aliens kept us in the same conditions as we keep our animals, I'm terrified to imagine what it would be like. If it's hard for you to imagine, too, below are a handful of scenarios to further assist in painting this horrendous picture.

Imagine a young teenage girl having just given birth, and her baby is taken away so that her breast milk can be harvested. While being milked until she runs dry, she's impregnated again, and then again, until she's physically spent and, essentially, useless, so she's then sent to become cheap burger meat (assuming aliens like burgers, too). Her daughters eventually join her in this cycle, but she never knows what happened to her sons.

Imagine young boys penned into fenced parking lots, eating nothing but protein bars and allowed no exercise, becoming the size of a grown man by only three years old so that they can be sent to slaughter sooner.

Imagine a mother giving birth in a tiny cage where she can't turn around, with only her breasts exposed for her child to suckle, before that child is taken away to be fattened up in a barn and sold for ribs.

Imagine thousands of babies living on the floor of a giant barn, on top of an infested build-up of their faeces, urine, and dead siblings. And when it's time for slaughter (at five weeks old), the workers come along and pick them up by any limb they can grab and sling them into crates.

Unfortunately, it's relatively easy (although deeply disturbing) to imagine this, because these are the common—and legal—practices of dairy cows, cattle feedlots, pigs, and broiler chickens.

What psychological conditions would we humans experience? Would we initially struggle to be free? Would we fight back, only to be repelled and treated more harshly? Would we then turn to in-fighting, cannibalism, madness, and hopelessness? And then would we eventually submit to a technologically superior race just because they're dominant? What would we think of them? What would justify their treatment of us? What argument would we use to convince them not to eat us? That we can think? That we can feel pain? That we just *exist*, and therefore we deserve to live our own lives?

This is the root of speciesism, in which one species places themselves at the top based on arbitrary characteristics and preferences, and justifies the treatment of others based on the misguided belief that one deserves more moral consideration than another[24]. Right now we're at the top, but it only takes a bit of imagination to put ourselves in the place of animals and realise that we wouldn't want it for ourselves.

We do these things to animals because our 'ingenious' and 'advanced' humanity allowed us to create the technology to do so. But it's that very same humanity that would be the reason we implore the aliens *not* to eat us, and so it follows

Chapter 2: Exploitation

then that our humanity should be the catalyst to not exploit non-human animals in the first place.

Ok. Let's take a breath. That was probably a bit more graphic and gruesome than I'd planned. However, it's important to note that the descriptions and details here are the standard, legally permitted treatments in countries like Sweden, Austria, the UK, Switzerland[25], and others that are considered 'the best in the world' for animal welfare standards. For more details on the reality of animal farming, you can (and should) check out the resource list at the end of the book.

~

Let's keep in mind that exploitation goes much further than what happens to the animals we turn into food. There's also the hidden cost of human exploitation—not by aliens (though they *are* out there, I'm sure of it!), but by the animal industry itself. Back in 1906, Upton Sinclair's *The Jungle* became an instant bestseller when it exposed the meatpacking industry as the most dangerous job in the world[26]. While it's a fiction novel, it *is* based on the real stories and experiences witnessed by the author when he went undercover in Chicago's meatpacking industry at the turn of the 20th century.

The story revealed underpaid migrants working in appalling conditions and treated as wage slaves. There was no sick pay, and the high risk of injury meant that workers easily lost their jobs. They worked long hours in disgusting conditions: standing all day in blood, guts, and poop; toilets right next to the processing line; and no hand washing facilities.

There are reports of rats, faeces, and human body parts making it into the meat that ended up being packaged for human consumption. From this startling exposé, the White House commissioned a report into the industry. Its inspectors verified these conditions, and even reported witnessing a pig carcass falling into a nearby toilet before being put back on the hook without being washed[27].

The Jungle caused such a stir that new regulations and laws were created to protect the people working in these terrible conditions. Within a year of its release, the White House had created the Meat Inspection Act and the Pure Food and Drug Act, the latter leading to the creation of the Food and Drug Administration (FDA). However, despite good intentions on the part of lawmakers and the public they were responding to, these new laws were hardly enforced. A 2004 Human Rights Watch report reviewed the one hundred years since *The Jungle* was released, and found that while wages and conditions improved during the 1940s and 50s, giving workers better wages than most manufacturing jobs, conditions began a steep decline backwards in the 1980s that continue to the present day[28].

Technological improvements and automation meant that there was less requirement for skilled workers. In some cases, companies closed entire plants and reopened down the road to get out from under the unions, so that they could hire migrant workers for less money and no rights. Automation also meant faster line speeds, placing even higher pressure on workers, and injuries today are now more than twice the manufacturing average. As of 2004, when the report was published, meatpacking employees receive on average 24%

Chapter 2: Exploitation

lower wages than other manufacturing jobs, even though Human Rights Watch has labelled it 'the most dangerous job in America'.

It's a similar story in Australia. Injury rates here are four times the national average, and some migrant workers are being paid less than $10 AUD an hour,* after mandatory company deductions for visas, accommodation, and furniture rental[29] (it would be nice if my employer decked out my condo, but I think I'd rather the money—and freedom—to make my own choices). Migrant workers dominate the landscape in Europe and the UK, too[30,31]. Working right alongside local employees, migrants receive around 50% less wages for the same job. Since they come through subcontracting firms, they have no sick pay, zero-hour contracts, and sham self-employment, which means that their rights aren't being observed. Many are brought in from overseas with the promise of a better life on an EU working visa, and they're forced to accept these conditions—if they lose their job, they become illegal immigrants. COVID also highlighted the problem in Europe's slaughterhouses. As migrant workers were unable to take a sick day without losing wages or potentially their job, these workplaces became hotspots for disease transmission, and many companies were exposed when they didn't have enough documentation for effective contact tracing. These terrible conditions are still allowed to flourish, because numbers of inspections and official regulators have been slashed in recent years, allowing companies to do their own thing basically without any oversight. One inspector per 10,000 workers[32]

---

* The Australian national minimum wage for adults in 2023 is $23.23.

is hardly enough to keep things in check.

Workers are exposed not only to high injury rates with the risk of losing fingers, limbs, and even their lives, but also to psychological damage. The trauma caused by electrifying, shooting, stabbing, and gassing animals to death over and over, sometimes as many as 175 birds or 18 pigs per minute[33,34], has an uncountable toll. In regular society, if someone were to stab a pet dog, we'd send them for psychological counselling and perhaps even lock them away from polite society, and yet slaughterhouse workers are expected to do this over and over, and there's no support for *them* when they come home to fit back into society. Desensitised to torture and death, this can lead to increased violence and mental illness. Reports in Australia show that aggression levels for slaughterhouse workers can be similar to people in prison, and that communities with a high proportion of slaughterhouses have increased rates for domestic violence, rape, and child abuse[29,35].

As with any industry, conditions differ from business to business. Many people I've spoken with affirm that these stories do match their experiences. Others assure me of the cleanliness (once you get past the unfathomable kill floor) but also tell me about terrible cultures with a boss who acts like Al Capone, and how the HR people are to be feared and not trusted. In any event, there's no denying the visual footage that brave undercover reporters risk their lives to expose in documentaries. And according to one source in Australia, even in abattoirs with an export license (where conditions are much more tightly regulated and sanitary, such as sterilising knives between each animal), the line speeds are still incessant

Chapter 2: Exploitation

and the working culture is still rife with low-paid migrant workers, high drug use, bullying, fighting, and even taking turns stabbing each other to claim workers comp (and no, that's not a joke or an exaggeration).

Similarly insidious is the exploitation of public trust. When Upton Sinclair wrote *The Jungle*, he intended it to be an exposé on the plight of the workers, but the public outcry was focused on all the gross stuff that ended up in their food and the fact that corporations try to get away with it. Slaughterhouse workers I've spoken with tell me about the pus they find daily in the animals as they cut them up. Sometimes there are giant nodules containing several litres that explode all over the worker. When this happens, the line is actually stopped, the clean-up crew comes in, the workers change clothes, and then the line starts up again. While these big ones are rare (one person I spoke with had only seen about four in his more than ten-year career), there are hundreds of 'little' ones they come across on a regular basis, containing only about 100ml of pus (that's about the size of a perfume bottle). To ensure these little bursts of extra flavouring don't end up in the rump of steak on our plate, they just cut around them (well, when they can *see* them. It's not like they have all day to thoroughly inspect each carcass—they've got quotas to meet).

And did you know that there's actually an acceptable limit of pus in milk? I'm really sorry if I've just made you spit out your sip of latte, but unfortunately, it's true. Dairy cows, genetically bred to produce increased amounts of milk, often suffer painful mastitis—an inflammatory infection of the udders—due to constant machine milking. This, along with other bacteria such as e-coli or listeria, regularly makes it into the cow's milk system and out through their udders. The USDA allows up to 750 million somatic[*] cells per litre; the EU allows 400 million; Australia has no limit[36]. Australia does appear to have an acceptable limit of faecal matter in milk, though; when Coles recalled a bunch of dairy products in 2016, it was because it found faecal bacteria 'in excess of quality standards'—not *some*, but *too much*[37]. While 750 million cells seem like a lot, in reality, Dr Michael Greger's calculations have worked out that it's probably not much more than a single drop of pus in a small cup of milk[38]. Still, if you watched someone take a syringe and slowly drop one dollop of pus into your glass, would you still drink it? Imagine that in your Milo.

The one that grosses me out the most (and I'll admit I *do* hope to pass that unsettling feeling on to you) is chickens and their 'faecal soup'[39,40]. Chickens are grown in giant barns where they're crammed together: walking, lying, and eating on top of their own excrement, and these barns are only washed out at the end of the four- to six-week growing cycle once the birds have been sent to slaughter. Being so close together is a hotbed for zoonotic diseases, as many studies have attested[41]. In addition to these conditions, chickens are selectively bred to grow as fast as possible, so they suffer from a variety of disease and injury such as organ failure, broken limbs, and sudden death syndrome. Due to all of this, many lives are lost each day. Barns commonly house between 10,000 and 40,000 birds, and while a daily task of the workers is to pick

---

[*] 'Somatic' refers to biological cells from our body.

Chapter 2: Exploitation

up and discard any dead birds they find, they obviously miss many, leading to more contamination from rotting carcasses. Estimates say that by the time the chickens are ready for slaughter, about half of them are diseased.

So how does a bit of poop get into all of them? As chickens are processed in the slaughterhouse, they go through the process of bleeding out; being dunked in boiling water to loosen feathers; the extraction of their internal organs; and finally, they're thrown into a giant chlorinated ice-water bath where they spin around to be washed and chilled. However, thousands are dumped in there together, with excrement, blood, and bacteria swirling around the water and soaking into their flesh for up to an hour. This is the water that's lovingly referred to as 'faecal soup'. If any chickens manage to survive their time in the barn and are still healthy, they're certainly contaminated by the time they come out of this chiller, with some studies finding up to 97% of consumer-packaged chicken testing positive for intestinal bacteria[41]. Yep, that's right: intestinal means poop.

There is, however, a cleaner option. An 'air' chiller exists, in which chickens don't mix together, preserving the clean status of the healthy ones[42]. Here's why chicken processors don't use it: besides water chillers being quicker and sometimes cheaper, chickens are sold based on weight, and marinating in the water chiller means that their meat soaks up more water content. This means that they're heavier (full of faecal soup), and so the farmer makes more money[43]. As usual, the almighty dollar is the main driver, not welfare (clearly of neither animals nor consumers).

Exploitation is also inherent anywhere else animals are used, such as for clothing, entertainment, and experiments. Did you know that leather isn't simply a by-product of the food industry? Leather can be a bigger economic driver of cow slaughter, especially in places like India. Beef is rarely eaten there, but they are nearly the largest global leather exporter in the world. Since cows are considered sacred in India, it means they are driven to find clandestine and hazardous ways around the laws, and treatments of animals and workers alike is usually a much lower standard than Western countries[44].

Some people may believe it's ethical to wear wool because sheep need to be sheared, but they only need to be sheared because we've bred them like that; natural sheep would drop their wool seasonally. Behind the scenes of 'entertainment' like circuses, aquariums, and zoos, animals can be cruelly treated, often encouraged with electric shocks to behave in unnatural ways and denied the ability to practice their natural habits[45]. And there's no special protection for babies: 'surplus' offspring are often discarded, like Marius the giraffe who was shot, autopsied, and fed to tigers in front of onlookers (including children) at Copenhagen Zoo in 2014[46,47]. In lab experiments, monkeys and rats are usually euthanised after an experiment, because they're now considered 'tainted' and not pure[48,49].

~

The major myth that has allowed all forms of exploitation to continue is the myth that eating animals is normal, natural, and necessary. Even if we *do* believe that eating animals is all fine and well, it's clear that there's nothing 'natural' about

Chapter 2: Exploitation

the way we use animals today. Yes, it's normal for lions to kill and eat other animals—it's also normal for dogs to greet each other by sniffing their butts, but you don't see anyone advocating that we adopt that behavioural trait. Even if lions killing deer in the wild *did* justify our own eating of animals, it wouldn't justify selectively breeding them with artificial insemination into canned hunting factories, using technology to confine and control their whole lives, and utilising modern medicine to keep them alive just long enough to be slaughtered by industrial machinery or gas chambers—and then eating them with a knife and fork.

Even for tribes around the world for which eating animals *is* a necessity for survival, they live in harmony with their environment and treat animals with reverence and responsibility. They understand the cycle of life and a balanced ecosystem, and they show empathy and gratitude for the gift of life their animals are providing. Many Indigenous belief systems revolve around reincarnation, and they regard animals with respect and equal status: in their next life the animals could become humans, or the humans might come back as animals. If they don't respect the animal's contribution to their life, or if they kill for pleasure and waste, then the animal spirit won't return and the people will starve[50].

Today's semi-nomadic Mongolian peoples, who live in the deserts and mountains, have limited opportunity for agriculture. For thousands of years, they've kept horses, sheep, and other animals who can eat the grasses that are unsuitable for humans, and the people survive from the milk, blood, and meat that the animals provide. As well, they use their bones and hides for clothing and shelter, and their dung for fuel[51].

While I have no inclination to join a wandering Mongolian tribe just to eat a bit of meat, I can appreciate they're doing what they need to do in order to survive.

In Australia, Aboriginal tribes have been shown to even *improve* species' numbers due to hunting. Their use of fire to clear land for hunting creates a mosaic pattern, with pockets of regrowth where species thrive. A study from 2013 shows how numbers of sand monitor lizards (a prime source of food) nearly double when traditional fire-hunting methods are used[52]. It's also telling that when native tribes were (forcibly) relocated from the desert to missions or pastoral ranches in the 1950s onwards, 10 to 20 species of desert animals went extinct within two decades, and more than 40 others went into steep decline. Aboriginal hunting methods are truly an example of a symbiotic relationship with the land and the animals they share it with. Similarly, there's evidence of early Homo sapiens in Sri Lanka who only hunted adult monkeys in their prime, thereby ensuring the sustainability of the animal population[53].

Today's 'hunting' methods have removed the respect, connection, and sustainability from the practice. It's no longer about survival and being custodians of the Earth—it's about cheap, mass-produced products, driven by profit, deceit, and exploitation. Unlike traditional tribes who live in harsh conditions and need animals for more than just food, the science is clear that in our Western world (where we have the luxury of choice), we don't need to eat animals for survival. We'll go into detail on the science of nutrition in the next chapter.

~

Chapter 2: Exploitation

Last year, I spent time at a friend's dairy farm. It's an idyllic rural country farm, and his parents had built the house from scratch before he was born. Though one of the smallest farms in his area, he has 94 heifers and knows them all by name. He also has dozens of chickens running around and laying eggs all over the place, and a couple of cats and dogs for good measure. During the day, the cows are out grazing somewhere in his many acres. He rotates the herd across day and night fields, bringing them in twice a day for milking and checking the status of their health. He keeps his cows much longer than the industry average of four to five years: many are eight or nine and still productive, and some of them are 16 or 17 years old. These older cows are 'retired', but he keeps them around because they're a good influence on the rest of the herd. About four years ago, he also stopped selling the male calves; he couldn't bear to 'put them on the truck' (yep—you know where). Chickens and roosters are free to roam, only coming indoors at night to keep the foxes away. He collects about a bucket of eggs every day and sells them at the local markets. It's as close to ethical and traditional animal husbandry as you could imagine.

Many of us know someone like this, or at least have a friend of a friend who's been to a beautiful, rural, small-town farm. Yes, animals are being raised for food, but the farmers are doing their best to give them a good life and treat them well in the meantime. This is what keeps the dream alive, and it's one of the justifications we use for continuing to eat animals. We hear the horrors of factory farms and say, 'Yeah, but it's not *all* like that…look at my friend's farm.' But do you get all your meat, eggs, and dairy from your friend's farm? Even if you do, does everyone else you know do, too? Logistically, this one farm can't produce the demand we require, and there's simply not enough land to have millions of farms like this one. It's also illegal to sell meat that you've slaughtered yourself (another way the industry controls their profits), so animals from these idyllic farms still need to go through the standard abattoir process to be sold to the public.

The demand for meat and dairy is what's driving the exploitation. In order to provide cheap meat and milk in sufficient quantities to keep up with supermarket orders (which themselves are driven by our weekly shop), the farmers have no other choice but to raise as many animals as possible, on as small a piece of land as possible, and get them to slaughter weight as quickly and cheaply as possible. Welfare isn't even a secondary consideration—it's much further down the list. The corporations who can do this best will outcompete the smaller operations, so those smaller operations get swallowed up, their ethical standards replaced by the more 'efficient' model. Like any business, they're simply responding to the consumer demand for 'more meat'. That's also the reason we see a lot more 'free range' and 'organic' products now: because the demand is there. Ultimately though, if we didn't eat it, they wouldn't make it.

~

When we look at being vegan with the plight of the animals in mind, it's clear to see why the idea of *not* being a 'perfect' vegan is hard to accept. For animals, the urgency is *right now*. Their lives are literally on the firing line, well before any climate change affects them.

Chapter 2: Exploitation

For the vegans who come into this lifestyle with animal rights as their main concern, it can be hard to imagine taking it slowly or putting our benefit of balanced meals and convenience over their right to live free. How can we justify drinking the milk of a mother whose baby was killed at birth, just because we don't like the taste of black coffee and 'This café has no alternative milks!'? The problem is that this is too big an industry to be affected by a handful of 'perfect' vegans.

If this was a niche dietary choice happening only in some parts of the world, such as dog meat, maybe it would be easier to stamp it out. However, we kill and eat 80 billion land animals globally every year[54]. Each chicken barn goes through about seven or eight non-stop cycles of 'hatch to harvest' every year. It's a worldwide industry that dominates our global foodscape, and most people don't even question it. It's going to take a lot of people making many reductionary choices in order to reduce the demand, slow down the industry, and eventually convert it into that niche dietary choice that's easier to eliminate and even easier to avoid.

If we want to help the animals, we need many reasons combining to join the cause. Environment is one, exploitation is another, and, as we'll see in the next chapter, it's also health. Most of us have been led to believe that we need to eat animals to survive, but this is simply untrue. These corporations have been using very clever marketing to convince us that we need their products, but science is revealing. The next chapter will explore the myths that have been perpetuated to make sure that we keep eating animals. For me, this deception is another reason to avoid the industry. No one likes being lied to.

CHAPTER 3: Marketing and Myths

The most common regret vegans have is not starting sooner, and once they begin learning about what's really going on, they just can't understand how so many others can continue to participate in something that's bad for their health, cruel to animals, and unsustainable to the environment. A huge part of the reason is because most people just don't know. The animal industry and the media don't want us to know about it, and they've intentionally kept us in the dark. Yes—*intentionally*. There's no financial incentive for them to show the truth, to cut through the confusion and lay it all out clearly. They benefit from obscurity and misinformation. They benefit from our ignorance.

This section is an integral part of the conversation, because when we take a step back and look at the whole picture, it's so unbelievably obvious.

Chapter 3: Marketing and Myths

To put it plainly, we've run out of time for the bullshit. Our planet is in peril, and rather than banding together so that we can save it, these giant corporations are still passing blame and pointing fingers. Like a toddler caught with paint on her hands, standing next to an 'artistically' decorated wall and saying, 'I didn't do it.'

However, thanks to the advance of technology, clever investigative journalism, smaller undercover cameras, increased consumer awareness, the wide reach of social media, and public demand for the truth, we're beginning to lift the lid. This section blows off that lid completely and exposes the stories we've been fed so that you can make up your own mind about whether this is an industry you want to keep supporting.

It All Started with Good Intentions

In the early 2020s, there were a lot of conversations around gender stereotypes, with the idea being that individuals are influenced by the media and people around them. We're guided in our likes and dislikes, without even realising it, right from the beginning of our birth. This then extends to the colours of the toys in the shops and the way teachers respond to us in school. As I was in my 30s in this decade, these conversations caused me to reflect and wonder: do I like what I like because I actually *like* it (hot pink toenail polish, dresses that twirl, talking about feelings) or is that what I've been conditioned to like because I'm a girl?

Whether we acknowledge it or not, we're a product of the world around us. Our dreams, hopes, fears, choice of job, choice of partner, what we think about others, and especially what we buy at the shops are all shaped by culture and society. You've probably heard sayings like, 'You are who your friends are' or 'You are the average of the five people you spend the most time with', right? And now there are even studies demonstrating that you're more likely to have the same interests and habits as the friends of your friends, even if you've never met them[1-3].

This isn't necessarily a bad thing, as it served an evolutionary purpose on the African savannah and helped us survive when fitting in was a matter of life or death. Plus, it's nice to have friends with the same passions with whom you can talk for hours, and, most of the time, it's just easier to do what everyone else is doing. But the risk is with relying on perceived authority figures who, whether they know it or not, might not be giving us the full truth—just like trusting the government's advice on healthy food choices. The food industry has big budgets to influence government decision makers, and they also employ clever marketing people who've figured out how to tap into these social influence tactics for public persuasion. Industry uses them (the government and the tactics) to shape the stories and myths all around us that we take for granted, and then we continue to perpetuate these myths through our buying choices. Because other people do what we do, too.

Did I eat meat because I wanted to? Or because that's what everyone else did? Was it because I was told that it's good for me, or because the alternatives weren't discussed? Or maybe my Dad just really nailed his BBQ steaks. (He did). I don't know if we'll ever know for sure where the line is drawn between our personal preferences and those of society's influence, but

Chapter 3: Marketing and Myths

we can at least educate ourselves and learn about the factors that are influencing us even when we're least paying attention. *Especially* when we're least paying attention.

~

When it comes to intensive animal farming—'factory farms', also known as 'concentrated animal feeding operations' (CAFOs)—it all started with good intentions. During the two world wars and the Great Depression, Western countries experienced food shortages, supply issues, and heavy rationing. Not surprisingly, the governments in these countries wanted to find a way to protect their people from experiencing these hardships in the future, and so they invested heavily in the agricultural industry in their own backyard. Subsidies in the form of guaranteed prices and confirmed quantities of orders were offered to protect farmers and increase production, such as in the Agricultural Act UK 1947 and the European Common Agricultural Policy[4,5].

Initially, it was seen as a great idea because farmers got wealthier and had job security, and the people had cheap and reliable sources of food. I'd be happy with that, too—on the surface. This protection for farmers, however, led to intensified production, larger corporations (and, of course, increased animal suffering that we explored in the previous chapter), and, with that, the desire to keep their profits, subsidies, and benefits. As these corporations got bigger, they looked for ways to drive up demand, increase their profits, and retain their power, and a huge part of that was to use their influence to position their products as desirable, affordable, and necessary.

In other words—marketing.

Today, we're eating an incredible amount of meat per person that we weren't eating only two generations ago[6]. Global meat production has more than quadrupled (4.77 times) since 1961, despite our population only doubling in that time. On average, the world is eating 20kg more meat per person in 2020 than in 1961. However, we can see a sharp contrast in developing countries compared to Western ones. In places like India, where the population is predominantly vegetarian, their consumption of meat has remained steady at an average of 4kg per person, but in the United States, where eating meat is a big part of the culture, annual consumption per person rose from 93kg in 1961 to 126kg in 2020. And China, which is rapidly becoming Westernised, started out similar to India in 1961 at less than 4kg per person, and has now multiplied consumption 15 times, currently averaging more than 60kg per person—a consumption rate more than double the world average[7]. What drove this rise in demand?

The intention of this chapter is to expose the forces that have been influencing us so that you can make your own decisions about what actions you choose to take. While not all myths and marketing are completely made up, they do tend to cherry pick their sources and highlight one perceived benefit while conveniently omitting the full story. It's like when I come home from a day at the shops and show my husband Phil the beautiful shoes I got at such an amazing sales price, while leaving the rest of my 'amazing deals' in the car until he's not looking. As marketing expert and entrepreneur Seth Godin says, 'Facts are irrelevant. What matters is what the consumer believes.' The purpose of marketing is to make you

Chapter 3: Marketing and Myths

believe that you want—and need—to consume their products.

Animal products have become so embedded in our diet that whole food groups have been reduced down to become synonymous in our minds with one essential part of our diet. Meat = protein, dairy = calcium, fish = omega-3s, and eggs = breakfast. That's not an accident—that's marketing. Just like when you hear Kleenex, you know we're talking about tissues; Hoover means vacuum cleaners; and Google has transposed into a verb that means to search for something online. While these brands may be well known and easy to access, they're not the only brand offering this product, and they may not even be the best. But they have clever marketing teams, they know how to win customers, and they spend a lot of money to retain market share. The animal industry is no different, and the following sections will expose the branding on top of the essential nutrients our bodies need so that you can make a choice about what you put in your shopping basket.

The myths and marketing I'll share with you are roughly grouped into three themes that underpin the justification of eating animal products—what Melanie Joy has called the Three Ns of Justification[76]—that it's natural, normal, and necessary.

Starting with necessity, the idea that 'we need to eat animals' seems like common sense because we used to eat animals for survival. In addition, a lot of the scientific research of the 20th century (when we developed all these fancy new measuring techniques) began to identify the benefits we get from animal flesh and secretions. The bit that's being left out of the story is that animals aren't the *only* source of these nutrients, and that when we eat animal products, we're getting a lot of potentially harmful ingredients along with the good stuff. We'll look at things like the protein myth, whether dairy is the best source of calcium, and how omega-3s became associated with fish. We'll explore how the government has been influenced (not so subtly) by the animal industry and the impact this has had on our dietary guidelines, and I'll share with you the truth of science that backs up healthy, plant-based food choices.

Next is the belief that eating animals is normal, that everyone does it, and that 'it's not that bad'. And if it was really bad, they'd get shut down, wouldn't they? That sounds like common sense, too; however, the animal agriculture industry knows that if it keeps the truth hidden from us, it's 'out of sight, out of mind' and we'll just accept it without question as a normal part of life. We'll explore the myth of 'not in my country', how humane-washing (a form of brainwashing that tries to convince us that animals for consumption are treated gently and with compassion) and libel laws are hiding the real truth of what goes on, and how welfare charities are only fighting for slightly better standards rather than eliminating suffering in total. Another protective mechanism these corporations employ is the constant barrage of lawsuits aimed at preventing plant-based companies from using 'meat' and 'milk' names for their food, and we'll see how this is potentially going to backfire on the animal industry.

The last group of myths is something that we tend to fall back on once we've opened our eyes to the reality that we don't need to eat animals, and see that it's actually pretty bad what the industry is doing. The myth of 'there's an ethical way to do it' is a desire to go back to the old natural ways of hunting or raising our own animals. It sounds idyllic, but it's

Chapter 3: Marketing and Myths

unfortunately not feasible. We'll explore how eating organic or local doesn't make much difference, how grass-fed cattle can be worse for climate change, and how the data shows there's just not enough land for us to continue eating anywhere near this volume of animal products in an old-fashioned, ethical, and natural way.

Throughout the following pages, I hope it's clear that I'm not telling you *what* to think: I'm asking you *to* think. You can make up your own mind whether this is something you can get behind, or whether you want to make an ethical stand for your own reasons. Look into the data, and don't take things at face value—especially the headlines on the evening news. Always ask yourself, 'Who's telling me this, and what do they have to gain from me believing them?'* In Part 3, I'll share some more tips for how to read scientific studies and critically evaluate the information of news articles. But for now, let's dive into the myths we've been fed.

Myth 1: We need to eat animals

Our Ancestors Ate Meat
The myth of our need to eat animals goes way back to our

---

*Even me! Why am I telling you this? What do I have to gain from you believing me and changing your eating habits? Question everything. But do keep in mind, however, that my ramblings here are entirely backed up by facts and science. Just saying.

evolution, where it's been proposed that once humans learned to cook and eat meat, our brains grew bigger, leading to our advancement as a species[8]. Although, maybe we overcooked it a bit, seeing as the derogatory term 'meathead' now means someone with *no* brains. Too much of a good thing? Anyway, the theory comes from finding remains of animal bones at ancient campsites from around the time that the human population began to expand. And that's true—those things did happen at the same time. But what's being left out of the picture is that it was fire itself that allowed us to cook *more* of all types of foods, including plant matter. Cooking makes food easier to digest so that we can extract more nutrients out of it, and we can spend less time chewing and more time exploring.

What science *does* show is the important role that carbohydrates play in the development of our brains[9], which would have been obtained from plants like roots and tubers (similar to potatoes, carrots, and beets), and not from meat. The reason we don't find plant matter at these ancient campsites is because it decomposes and goes back into the soil, so there's simply no evidence of food scraps from plants.

One thing that's important when it comes to scientific research is the concept that 'absence of evidence is *not* evidence of absence'; just because there's no evidence of plant food remains, this isn't evidence that it never existed. There's definitely evidence that we ate meat—that's not in question—but positioning it as the sole driver of the evolution of our brain and species is a case of cherry picking the facts[10,11].

Chapter 3: Marketing and Myths

Protein

One of the most pervasive myths of eating meat is that we need to consume it for protein. Well, protein certainly *is* essential—no arguments there. It's used by every cell in our body to do basically everything, including growth, digestion, repairs and maintenance, transporting nutrients, and more. Each of the thousands of different proteins in our body are comprised of 20 amino acids, nine of which are considered 'essential' because our bodies don't make them internally, so we need to get them from food.

The myth is that while animal meats are a 'complete' source of protein, plant sources are apparently not. It's true that meat does contain all nine of these proteins in good quantities; however, every single plant food *also* contains all nine essential amino acids, just in varying quantities[12]. You may have heard some plants, like soy and quinoa, referred to as 'complete' sources of protein, but what that means is that they contain amounts of all nine in similar quantities to animal products rather than an unbalanced mix. It's such a pervasive myth that it's still common to come across vegan health food articles talking about plants that are 'complete' and noting which ones you need to combine to make your meal a proper, nutrient-full one. In reality, it's more about balance.

Here's one of the things I love about how clever our bodies are: for thousands of years, cultures around the world have been eating common food pairings that make balanced proteins. Without knowing the science, we eat them because they taste good together, and that's our body's way of letting us know what we need. Some of these pairings include rice and beans (rice is low in lysine, which beans are high in),

Indian Dahl (lentils and rice), or hummus (beans) and pita (grains)[14]. The good thing is that we don't even need to eat 'balanced' proteins in every meal, as long as throughout the day we're eating a variety of plant foods from legumes (that's beans and lentils), whole grains, nuts, and seeds. It's simple to do, and these things will give you all the protein you need.

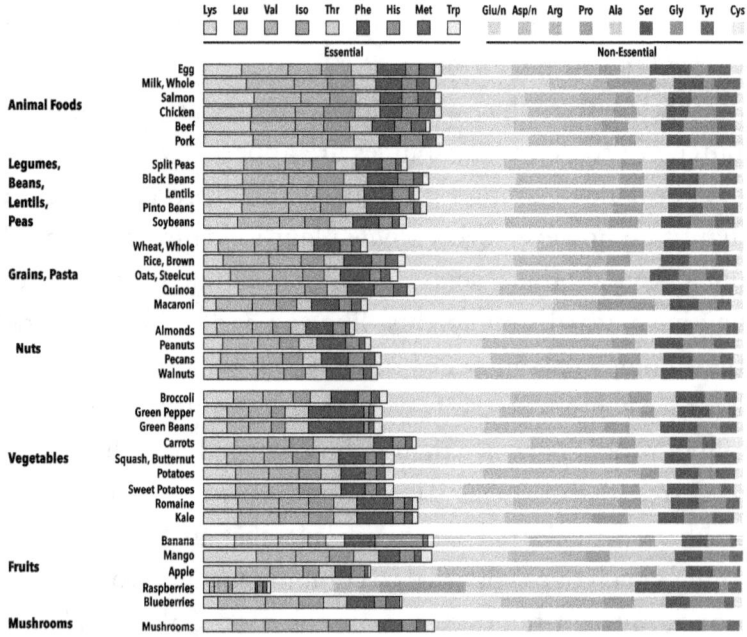

Figure 10: All Essential Amino Acids in All Food Types, Just in Varying Proportions[13]

One tactic of the meat industry is to demonise soy, and for years they've been perpetuating a myth by insinuating that soy is 'feminising' (due to its high estrogen content) and

Chapter 3: Marketing and Myths

that it causes breast cancer. Soy is a well-known 'complete' protein (in other words, it has a similar amino-acid balance to animal meats), and such a versatile bean is a great alternative for those on plant-based diets. From this incredible little bean, we get tofu, tempeh, edamame, milk, soy sauce, textured vegetable protein (TVP), and heaps of other cool stuff. The theory is that if the animal industry demonises a vegan's main viable protein alternative, it makes it harder to be vegan and more likely for vegans to return to meat for health reasons or convenience or both[15]. But are their claims true? (Spoiler alert: negative.)

The fear of soy being associated with breast cancer comes from studies that implanted human breast tissue into rats, who were then fed an isolated part of soy called isoflavones. This is so far removed from the way we consume soy in our diet that it's kind of laughable. For a start, humans are not rats. Additionally, our breast tissue doesn't need to be implanted into our bodies (pretty sure it grows naturally for us, unless I was mysteriously needled in the night by the boob fairy when I was 12), and we consume whole plants as part of a varied diet instead of only one isolated compound, and certainly not in the ginormous quantities used in animal trials. Studies have also shown that rats metabolise these compounds less effectively than humans, thereby increasing their risk of tumours[16]. When we look at studies on real people, soy is *actually* shown to improve health outcomes and reduce the risk of some cancers[17,18]. And the feminising thing? The estrogen in soy is actually *phyto*estrogen (phyto = plant-based), which has a much weaker effect on the human estrogen receptors in our hormone system. Nor does soy have any impact on testosterone levels: a meta-analysis combined the results of clinical studies between 2010 and 2020 and found that soy, in any of its forms, had no significant impact on any male reproductive hormones[19]. Soy isn't evil, nor is it a wonderbean that solves all health problems: it's just another plant that can happily be consumed in a varied diet.

Another myth regarding protein is that animals are a better-quality source of protein, but again, the reason for 'better' is cherry picking key features. One feature they call out is that animal meat contains high quantities of all nine essential amino acids, but it's also promoted that animal proteins are easier to digest. And this is indeed true, but the difference is only about 10-20% and negligible unless you suffer from protein deficiency (in which protein makes up less than 10% of calories, and this is a very rare condition, mostly affecting those living in extreme poverty)[20]. Animal proteins come with bad things like saturated fats and cholesterol, whereas plant proteins come with fibre, good fats, vitamins, and minerals. Even though animal meats are a good source of iron, protein, zinc, and B12, they're not the *only* source of those nutrients, and they're missing tons of essential micronutrients. And it also doesn't negate the fact that the World Health Organisation and Cancer Council have advised that processed meats are 'carcinogenic to humans' and that red meat is 'probably carcinogenic' due to its associations with several types of cancers[21,22]. In addition, studies comparing animal protein to plant sources demonstrate an overall higher quality of life and lower disease risk with plants[23,24].

Plant proteins have also been demonised because of phytates[25], which are naturally occurring compounds in plants

Chapter 3: Marketing and Myths

that are designed to protect themselves from bacterial infections and being eaten by insects. Pretty cool, right? Kind of like our own immune systems. However, by doing this, they can bind to other vitamins and minerals to reduce their absorption in our bodies. The good news is that this is predominantly an issue in cases of poverty where the diet is limited in variety and high in starch, and it's also known that the effect of phytates can be reduced by cooking. Conversely, studies in humans show that phytates, when consumed as part of a varied diet, actually contribute to overall good health by slowing digestion, preventing sharp blood-sugar spikes, and providing antioxidant benefits[20,26,27].

So then, you can clearly see that while animal meat does contain high amounts of protein, the whole story isn't being told, as meat comes with many unwanted side effects, and plants are shown to be better for overall health. Plants for the win in the protein competition.

Dairy

When we think of calcium, we think of milk, right? I grew up, as I'm sure you did, knowing that for strong bones, we should be drinking milk. But where did this come from? The truth is that calcium *is* essential for strong bones, and it's also true that dairy products like milk *are* a high source of calcium. However, this is another example of the way marketing pulls out one key benefit of the product and simplifies the story. Calcium isn't the only thing we need for strong and healthy bones, and dairy isn't the only source of calcium (and not even the *best* source, as we'll see).

We can easily get calcium from a range of nuts, leafy

greens, tofu, and fortified plant milks. While dairy is a high source of calcium, studies have shown that we only absorb about 25% of calcium in these products[28]. Veggies like kale and broccoli actually have about double the absorption rate of calcium compared to dairy. Additionally, although calcium is important for bone health, there are many additional factors that are essential for strong bones, such as vitamin D, potassium, protein, and even weightlifting. Therefore, focusing solely on dairy consumption for the calcium benefits will leave many things unaddressed, and it could increase the risk of bone diseases such as osteoporosis. Maybe drop the baby cow growth formula in favour of some broc and a barbell? Definitely worth considering, at least.

Although the common story we're told is that dairy consumption can prevent osteoporosis, this bone-weakening disease has many contributing factors, including smoking, sedentary lifestyle, and even having more pregnancies—not just the amount of calcium consumed. Several large longitudinal studies, following thousands of people over decades, couldn't demonstrate a reliable connection between drinking milk and a reduction in fractures[29-31]. In fact, it can be demonstrated that countries with the highest dairy intake also have the highest rates of hip fractures, although this may not be linked purely to calcium. It's more likely due to their higher latitudes and longer winters, meaning that their bones don't get adequate vitamin D*. Other studies have shown that high intakes of dairy, even though still below the recommended three to four servings per day, have also been associated with an increased

---

* Our best source of vitamin D is the sun. We actually photosynthesise it—just like plants do!

Chapter 3: Marketing and Myths

risk of prostate cancer[32].

So why do we all think that milk is good for us? Marketing, perhaps? Of course! Alissa Hamilton, in her book *Got Milked?*, makes a detailed exploration of the dairy industry and its deceptions, and Mark Kurlansky's *Milk!* explores its history[33,34].

Here's a little summary for you. Starting back in the 1800s, milk carried a negative image, due in part to unsanitary conditions that spread diseases like typhoid, and also to the cheap 'swill milk' that was produced by distillery dairies and had an unappetising, sickly, blue fluid. Unscrupulous manufacturers dressed it with chalk, flour, molasses, and other substances, and then sold it to the unwitting public as 'Pure Country Milk'. Regrettably, thousands of children died every year during this period, but the government did little to intervene. And the dairy industry continued to promote it as a healthy drink, especially as the industrial revolution saw many mothers going to work, and cow's milk became a convenient substitute for breastmilk.

During the wars of the 20th century, powdered milk was in high demand for soldiers overseas. However, the fluid milk was a leftover by-product, and farmers hesitated to produce so much powdered milk if their fluid was just going to waste. So the ever-clever dairy industry came up with the school milk program, mandating that milk be provided with school lunches, and voilà—farmers had a reason to produce high quantities of milk for the war. Many farms converted to pure dairy to help with supply, but after the war when demand dropped, supply remained high, meaning prices fell, and so, caving to union pressure, governments stepped in.

Instead of encouraging farmers to make a different

product, governments around the world used taxpayer subsidies to guarantee prices, place minimum orders, and help with marketing campaigns[35]. This is where we saw the introduction of dietary guidelines recommending four glasses a day, as well as 'Got Milk?', one of the most popular campaigns ever (if a celebrity wasn't photographed with a milky stache, were they even famous?). National governments even had 'buy back' schemes, in which they'd buy any excess supply—so *of course* farmers continued to produce huge quantities of milk, cheese, butter, and other products that there was no market for: they knew the government would buy their excess stock. This led to crazy things like 'butter mountains' and 'cheese caves' that are still going on today. Honestly—google it!

Alongside influencing our governments, dairy marketing is a huge industry. While part of the game is making deals with restaurants, manufacturers and fast food chains, to create inventive products that contain more cheese[36] (like McDonalds' new 'cheesy range' that has a deep-fried cheese patty inside the burger, and comes with a side of mozzarella sticks), dairy industry boards mostly focus on the story that milk is essential. In Australia in the 1990s, Dairy Australia picked up on the osteoporosis endemic that was predicted. Ignoring all other contributing factors, they took one of them—calcium—and ran widespread campaigns aimed at getting teens and young adults to drink milk again[37]. Marketing is even being promoted as research and science, like this one:

As reported by Media Watch[38], a 2023 newspaper article claimed that a new study *by Dairy Australia* found 97% of Australians aren't getting enough dairy. In the article, a nutritionist *from Dairy Australia* backs up the claims, and in

Chapter 3: Marketing and Myths

the photo supporting the article, the dad with two daughters happily holding their glasses of milk and sporting fun milk moustaches is *a member of Dairy Australia's marketing team*.

(I used italics to highlight the details that were conveniently *left out* of the article.)

When Media Watch tried to verify the claim of 97%, it wasn't found in the study itself, and it took correspondence with Dairy Australia to confirm there was a discrepancy in how the number was reported—it actually related to the percentage of people who are *unaware of their daily requirements*, NOT those who weren't *meeting* their requirements. Whether or not an intentional mistake, most of us hear the news and latch onto the headline, and very rarely do corrections or apologies make it onto the same platform. This is why, in Part 3, I'll cover how to decipher marketing from science.

To be clear, and from a health perspective, I'm not saying that dairy needs to be avoided completely (unless, of course, you're lactose intolerant, then it's the devil). Dairy can certainly be helpful in meeting some nutritional requirements in an otherwise deficient diet, and the sanitation issues are mostly fixed up these days. But it's not *essential*, and our belief that it *is* comes down to *marketing*. So while dairy may indeed be high in calcium, we now know it's not our only source. We also know that it may come with a host of other risks that aren't present when consuming higher-quality calcium from plants. Our demand for dairy products has been influenced by clever marketing and government recommendations (themselves heavily influenced by industry lobbying, which we'll explore soon), yet we don't see this because the myths around dairy are so pervasive and ingrained in our culture.

Fish = Omega-3s?

I'm sure you've heard that fish are an excellent source of omega-3s—the 'good fats' that are essential for things like heart health, brain function, and keeping our cell membranes strong. And while it's true that fish have a high concentration of omega-3s, fish also have high concentrations of mercury, microplastics, and PCBs (industrial chemicals)[39,40]. Why? Because oceans are the dumping ground of all our human waste. Not just our bodily waste and bath water, but all the pesticides we spray on our crops, chemicals we use in manufacturing, radioactive waste…no matter where we dump it, rainwater and rivers wash it all out towards the oceans. Fish all around the world are infected with our waste products, and due to bio accumulation it stays in their bodies until we eat them, and then it stays in *our* bodies. While we're not exactly glowing green from all the radioactive waste we've absorbed, we may well be infusing our cells with a smorgasbord of toxins that wreak untold havoc on our health. The good news is, like dairy with its calcium, fish are not our only—or best—source of omega-3s.

There are many plant-based sources of omega-3s, such as chia seeds (delicious in yoghurt), flaxseeds (grind 'em up for your smoothie), and walnuts (chop 'em up and sprinkle on top of your salad), but the best place to get omega-3 is the same place fish get it from. 'What's that?' I can hear you wondering. 'Fish have to *get* omega-3s from *elsewhere?*' Yep, that's right—fish don't manufacture omega-3s: they absorb it from the algae (plants) they eat. Taking a daily algae oil supplement instead of eating fish or taking fish oil means that you get all the benefits of omega-3s without the added toxins supplied through fish as the middlemen.

Chapter 3: Marketing and Myths

In the effort to convince us that we need to eat fish, the industry is also painting them as a fresh, healthy source of nutrients. And they're *literally* painting them: did you know that farmed salmon fillets are actually a dullish grey? A colouring pigment is added to their feed to dye their flesh, and fish producers can choose from a colour palette depending on how pink they want it[41]. Mind. Blown. Documentaries like *Eating Our Way to Extinction*[42] and *Seaspiracy*[43] expose some of the harmful and unethical activities involved in both wild and farmed fish. Fish are hardly the clean food choice that marketers would have us believe.

Other Nutrients of Note

We explored how one of the first things a vegan is usually asked is, 'Where do you get your protein?', because protein is the most commonly associated nutrient that we get from meat (and most people aren't aware of how abundant plant-based protein sources actually are). However, there are several other vitamins and minerals that come neatly packaged in animal flesh, and the animal agriculture industry will often try to convince us that the only way we can get these is by consuming their products. So below are a couple of the key ones, and the places where you can easily obtain them on a plant-based diet.

(Please note that I've extensively researched this for my own needs, and I've spent time working with nutritionists to make the right choices for myself. Any information provided is purely from my own experience, and while I have had this section reviewed and approved by my accredited dietitian

from Plant Nutrition and Wellness, *please seek professional advice from your doctor or a dietitian when adjusting your diet, including supplements.)*

Vitamin B12[44,45]
This is one of those vitamins that we used to easily get from our food. B12 is made by bacteria in the soil when cobalt is present, so for most of our history we got plenty by consuming unwashed vegetables and drinking river water. But because we now wash our food and filter our water to avoid other harmful bacteria—which is a good thing—our steady alternative source of B12 is usually animal flesh.

But just like fish not manufacturing omega-3s directly, cows and other animals only manufacture B12 when they've ingested the right nutrients from the soils around the plants they eat out of the ground, and even that isn't enough anymore. For one reason, factory farming means that animals have limited exposure to soils in their lifetime, and even when they do graze naturally, monocropping has basically destroyed the nutrients like cobalt that microbes need to make B12 in the first place. Because of this, most animals are supplemented with B12*, so when we consume their flesh, we're getting B12 from the supplements *they* were given.

The best way to get B12 is to take a supplement yourself and cut out the middle mammal. In fact, doctors advise most people (especially those over 50) to take a B12 supplement

---

* It's been claimed that around 90% of all B12 supplements that are manufactured are given to animals, but there doesn't seem to be an industry report with this figure in. However, even a quick, cursory search of animal feed products shows most of them to be fortified with B12 or cobalt.

regardless of their diet. Without B12, we don't have enough red blood cells (which carry oxygen to our muscles, tissues, and organs), so we risk fatigue, weakness, memory loss, nausea, and other ongoing symptoms. I have a very simple B12 spray that goes under the tongue, and I spritz it into my system once or twice a week. It tastes like raspberries, and that suits me just fine.

Iron[46]

This mineral is essential for building strong red blood cells and for the normal function of cells and hormones, and a deficiency of it could leave you tired, confused, and short of breath. It's a myth that iron only comes from bloody red meat. There are two types of iron: heme (which comes from animal products) and non-heme (which comes predominantly from plants). Non-heme is not as well absorbed as heme, but that doesn't mean it doesn't work; it just takes a bit of planning. Iron is plentiful in plants like lentils, whole grains, nuts, seeds, and leafy greens, and when eaten alongside vitamin C (as in capsicum, tomatoes, or citrus fruits), it increases the absorption rate. I eat a lot of lentils, and I usually make a casserole with a tomato base and then add in red capsicum as one of the veggies. Another way of easily getting a good serve is my daily kale (iron) and mango (vitamin C) smoothie.*

Selenium[47,48]

I'd never heard of this mineral until I went vegan, but now I

---

* I've recently been experimenting with rainbow chard (also known as silverbeet) instead of kale, which has a surprising and refreshing flavour. But any dark leafy green will do.

know it's one of those essential ones that we need to get from food—it powers our metabolism, boosts our immune system, protects against heart disease, and supports brain function. Those eating meat or dairy on a daily basis will be getting enough selenium, but the highest source is actually Brazil nuts. I have a bag of these in my kitchen and I take one a day, just like popping a pill (but please do chew it; they're huge nuts. Well, technically they're seeds, but I doubt we'll ever catch on to calling them that, so 'nuts' it is). Selenium toxicity is an actual thing to be aware of, though, so it's not recommended to eat handfuls every day. Often, I'll skip several days of my 'pill' in its whole form, and instead have a few chopped Brazil nuts in my yoghurt or as a topping for my salad, or mix them into my homemade protein balls.

Iodine[49]

This one's a mineral that's essential for healthy thyroid function—without it, we risk infertility, slow metabolism, and poor brain function. During pregnancy, iodine deficiency can result in miscarriage, stillbirth, birth defects and developmental delays. We get it in our diet through seafood, dairy products, and iodised salt. I never considered it an issue until I realised that we were using a lot of these fancy new salts, like Himalayan pink salt or sea salt. While delicious, they don't naturally contain iodine, which would have to be added to them. However, I can easily buy iodized *rock* salt from the shops; it's right there next to all the other ones, and I check the labels of my bread and wraps to make sure they use iodized salt (and most of them do).

Chapter 3: Marketing and Myths

Zinc[50-52]

This powerhouse mineral is necessary for almost 100 functions in our body, including creating DNA, growing cells, building proteins, healing wounds, and supporting our immune system. The reason it's mentioned as a risk for vegans is because while it's found in high concentrations in plant foods, it may have lower bioavailability due to the presence of phytates. As we examined earlier, cooking is one way to reduce the impact of phytates, as is sprouting, fermenting, and soaking. However, studies show that vegans only need to increase their zinc intake by about 50%, and since it's a trace mineral, that's really not a lot, and so vegans are at no greater risk of zinc deficiency than the general population. Another way our bodies are incredible is that over time, they learn to increase our extraction from zinc sources, essentially overriding the lower bioavailability. Amazing, right? I'm constantly suprised by the clever machinery we've come to this Earth in. High sources of plant-based zinc include lentils, tofu, mushrooms, quinoa, pumpkin seeds, and pine nuts (add some kale and cherry tomatoes to that and you've got yourself a delicious salad).

Creatine[53]

You might've only heard of this stuff in reference to body builders—that's certainly all *I* thought it was for. I used to think (while rolling my eyes) that it was what the guys took before they hit the gym so they could get bulging, ripped muscles*. And yes, creatine does increase muscle fibre and energy stores so that we can go harder for longer, but creatine is actually important for everyone, especially those who don't eat meat.

---

* There's those gender stereotypes again!

It's not considered an 'essential' amino acid because our body does manufacture it, but usually not in enough quantity. We make about half in our bodies and get the other half from food—more specifically, from meat. So for those who *don't* eat meat, supplementing with creatine can also help with muscle recovery and reducing damage after exercise, and it also supports optimal brain function like memory and intelligence. Creatine monohydrate is one of the most highly studied supplements, and there've been no ill effects found to date. I personally take a dose with water every day, right before I have my pre-gym protein snack. My husband puts a dose in his water bottle in the morning or adds it to his protein shake. And while creatine isn't essential, I definitely wanted to dispel the myth that surrounds it. As for whether or not you'll be rocking massive delts and pecs by supplementing it, only time and a gym membership will tell. In the meantime, it's still an important amino to have in our systems (even for those of us who prefer yoga and a walk).

The Truth About Plant-Based Diets

The pervasive and resounding myth that most of us have grown up believing is that we need to eat animals to survive, but the science is showing that this just isn't the case.

One of the best sources for this is Simon Hill's book *The Proof is in the Plants*[54]. Highly detailed and extensively referenced, Hill is my go-to guy for getting to the truth and exploring the nuance of the studies and what they actually mean. I highly recommend his book and checking out his podcast and YouTube, where he regularly debunks myths, provides the other side of the story, and explains things in plain English but with fully backed-up science and evidence. Have a look at his video debunking the phytate issue, too[55].

The evidence for plant-based diets comes from many sources, but one report that's referenced a lot is the EPIC study, which has been following more than 500,000 people from ten European countries since 1999 to evaluate their quality-of-life outcomes based on diet. The EPIC-Oxford cohort was a UK branch of this study, which specifically looked at vegan and vegetarian diets compared to omnivores and is one of the largest studies of its kind in the world. Unequivocally, this study demonstrated that those who ate predominantly whole food plant-based (WFPB) diets lived longer, had lower rates of disease and death, and even the 'unhealthy' vegans had better outcomes than regular Western-style meat eaters with lower heart disease, cancer, and diabetes[56,57].

We see further evidence for the healthy outcomes of eating mostly plants when we look into the 'Blue Zones'—these are five regions around the world with the most centenarians (people over 100 years old) who aren't merely alive, but also thriving, active, and productive members of the community[58]. Ikaria in Greece, Loma Linda in California, Sardinia in Italy, Okinawa in Japan, and Nicoya in Costa Rica are geographically dissimilar, but they have a few key things in common. Aside from social factors like contribution to the community and having close relationships, the thing that stands out—the thing they do all day, every day—is what they eat. The diet in these Blue Zones is predominantly plant-based, comprised of whole grains, lentils, beans, nuts, seeds, vegetables, and fruits. They do eat a small amount of meat and dairy, but it's no more than 5-15% of total calories, in much smaller amounts per serving, and only a couple of times a month. It's definitely not the Western diet model, in which meat is the star of the show and comprising 50-80% of the plate for every meal.

One of the reasons people say they can't be vegan (or struggle to stay vegan) is that they think they can't be healthy without animal products. I want to be clear, however: this actually *is* the case for some people. We each have variations in our genetic make-up that make us intolerant to certain foods, and I've spoken to many ex-vegans who've had to reintroduce meat for one reason or another. But for the vast majority of people without any unique health complications, WFPB diets are the healthiest way to eat, not only for our bodies but for the planet as well.

A huge study in 2019 by the EAT-Lancet Commission explored how we would feed ten billion people on the planet, taking into consideration the boundaries of personal health and planetary health, using scientific targets for sustainable food production. It took a holistic approach, aiming to find the ultimate diet that met our health needs and the needs of our planet, such as limiting biodiversity loss, water usage, and GHG emissions. After modelling various types of diets, it ultimately found that the WFPD diet—the healthiest one for our bodies—was also the best option to fit within our sustainable planetary boundaries. If you want to follow the best diet for the sustainability of the planet, this study explains why plant-based is the way to go[59,60].

Interestingly, the EAT-Lancet Commission's healthy planetary diet doesn't recommend 100% plant-based: it allows for up to 12% of calories to come from animals. This is good news for the meat lovers out there: the issue of animal

Chapter 3: Marketing and Myths

exploitation aside, it's not going to kill you to have a small amount of good quality meat from ethical sources. To date, there's no science that shows any benefit of being 100% plant-based—the benefits come from 85% and above. Therefore, if you were to base your decision purely on health reasons (again, not considering the exploitation factor) it's not to say that we can never eat meat, just that it has to be significantly reduced and seen as a rare treat (or perhaps medium rare, depending on your palate).

But the Government Says...

If the science is so clear and we don't actually *need* to eat animals, why is no one talking about it? Well, *some* people are. Most of the dietetics associations around the world have made clear statements that a properly planned vegan diet is healthy for all stages of life, including pregnancy, infants, adolescence, old age, and even athletes[61]. David Attenborough, in his 2020 biographical documentary *A Life on Our Planet*, says, 'We must change our diet. The planet can't support billions of meat eaters.'[62] And, as we uncovered way back in our introduction, the United Nations has been including this recommendation in its reports since 2006. Even Arnie, a world-renowned champion bodybuilder, is touting a plant-based diet now[63].

So why are most governments still telling us to include meat, eggs, and dairy for essential nutrients as part of a balanced diet? It comes down to the simple—and somewhat sinister—truth: large corporations are protecting their profits. Over the years, they've invested heavily in driving up consumer demand for their products, buying out smaller holdings and extracting subsidies and support from governments. They've created a billion-dollar industry that's worth more than most countries*[64,65]: it's no wonder they don't want to lose that. In addition, they've been taking advantage of the gap left by the fact that doctors receive little to no compulsory nutrition education in their degree[66] (most four-year degrees might have one unit on the subject), and to fill that gap, they instead use marketing money to create self-serving dietary advice for the public.

The fact is, buying influence is how things get done. All around the world, industries that represent animal products have used lobbying and sponsorship to fund misleading science[67], buy into school nutrition programs, and influence dietary guidelines, convincing us that a balanced diet is not complete without meat, dairy, and eggs.

Even as recently as when this book went to press, documents were leaked that demonstrate how the meat and dairy industries are able to influence the United Nations' recommendations[68]. In March 2023, the IPCC released the Synthesis Report of their sixth Assessment Report for climate change. The Assessment reports are comprehensive and detailed, covering several years of reporting and scientific findings, and the Synthesis is a brief document outlining the key features, written in accessible language, that governments use to make policy decisions. Leaked documents show that their draft Synthesis included a statement about 'plant-based diets' being able to reduce GHG emissions by up to 50%

---

* In 2021, the global meat industry was worth nearly $900 billion USD. Only 19 countries (out of almost 200) have a higher yearly GDP. When you combine it with the dairy market value, that figure doubles[64,65].

Chapter 3: Marketing and Myths

compared to standard Western diets. However, countries like Argentina and Brazil, influenced by successful lobbying from their meat industries, rejected the draft and proposed alternative wording. The final version has now removed any mention of 'plant-based', and refers instead to wishy-washy terms like 'sustainable diets'. But for those who have the time and technical understanding to read the full report, the findings clearly speak to the huge planetary destruction coming from the meat and dairy industries.

The influence of industry is also clear in the health recommendations coming from our governments. The United States Department of Agriculture (USDA) produces the healthy dietary guidelines for its citizens, yet it's also the body responsible for dairy promotion, or, in other words, getting more people to consume more dairy[69]. The committee for the US guidelines is also predominantly made up of people who have associations with food manufacturers, and the publication of the guidelines has a history of changing its recommendations due to lobbying by bodies such as the meat industry[70,71]. In the UK, the Agriculture & Horticulture Development Board (AHDB), created by meat and milk levy bodies and funded by farmers, co-created the UK dietary guidelines and has also spent money lobbying the British Dietetic Association[72]. The British Nutrition Foundation, a charity that provides free nutrition education in schools, delivers this training in partnership with the AHDB, a primary sustaining member of the charity ('sustaining member' means that the charity receives substantial funds from industry)[73]. Australia's latest dietary guidelines were written in 2013 by the Dietitians Association of Australia (DAA), at a time when it was sponsored by Meat

& Livestock Australia, Nestlé, Dairy Australia, and the Egg Nutrition Council[74]. Can you see the conflicts of interest here?

It's not all bad news, though: the DAA changed its policy in 2019 and no longer partners with any food manufacturing or food industry associations, so hopefully the new Australian guidelines in 2023 will be influence-free. Canada, too, seems to have escaped this trap, as its newest dietary guidelines have been produced under scientific and dietitian advice, without any influence from industry[75]. Instead, following the science, they advise eating whole grains, fruits, and vegetables, and choosing plant-based proteins most often. Contrary to 22 states in the US that have milk as their state's official drink, Canada says *water* should be the drink of choice for everyone, and it's now completely removed dairy as a food group. It also specifically calls out the lesser environmental impacts of plant foods compared to animal foods, and warns consumers to 'be aware of food marketing'. When we know that human beings are biologically the same in Canada as they are over the border in the US or across the world in Australia, and that we all therefore have the same nutritional requirements no matter where we live, it's clear to see where the influence of industry plays out.

At this point, you might be thinking that you as an individual have no power to do anything when it comes to these huge multi-national, billion-dollar corporations. But let's think about it: Where does all this money for lobbying and influence come from? It comes bit by bit, $11 here and $2.95 there, every time we shop at the supermarket for a steak or a carton of eggs. When we buy the products of these companies, we're not only giving them profits—we're giving them *power*.

Chapter 3: Marketing and Myths

We think that we're giving governments power when we vote for them, but we're giving corporations way more power when we buy their products, and then they use *our* money to buy government officials. It's not an understatement to say that we vote with our wallet. The real power is in our hands.

And the good news is that the façade is beginning to crumble. Yes, the meat industries still lash out in protest against any plant-based advertising, but we now have more access to information. We can research for ourselves and see both sides of the story, without simply being persuaded by TV ads, controlled by those with the most money and lobby power.

Myth 2: It's not that bad

Humans Eat Animals

Ok, so it may not be necessary, but it's at least *normal* for humans to eat animals, isn't it? All the humans do it, all around the world. That's true, but have you ever thought about why we eat certain animals and not others? In the Western world, why do we eat cows but not dogs? Some parts of Asia happily eat dogs. Why does India not eat cows? Most of the Middle East doesn't eat pigs, but Aussies love some pork on the fork. Some countries in Europe eat horses, but not the UK.[*] Most of us don't question drinking milk and eating cheese made from a cow, but would have to take a minute before trying,

---

[*] Unless by accident. I was living there during the 2013 'horse meat scandal' where horse meat was 'accidentally' mixed in with products labelled 'beef'. Even still, horsemeat was regularly eaten in the UK until about the 1930s, but now they say 'neigh'.

say, pig's cheese (tempted?), and most grown men are even grossed out by human breast milk, if that episode of Friends is anything to go by, and I'd say that it is. Have you ever stopped and wondered why? I loved understanding the psychology behind this, and it was Melanie Joy's detailed exploration of the topic in her landmark book *Why We Love Dogs, Eat Pigs, and Wear Cows: An Introduction to Carnism*[76] that finally caught my attention and launched my own vegan journey.

Dr Joy coined the term 'carnism', which is the ideology in opposition to the belief system of 'veganism'. In fact, she wrote her whole PhD thesis on the topic. She explained that there really wasn't a term that described the opposite of veganism. 'Meat eater' is the commonly used expression, but that only describes what someone eats rather than what they believe, and words like 'omnivore' or 'carnivore' are actually scientific terms relating to biological processes of digestion[*]. And as we know, veganism is more than a diet: it's a way of life underpinned by a belief system that it's wrong to exploit animals or consume their products.

The opposite ideology—that it's *okay* to exploit animals and consume their products—didn't have a name because it's so pervasive that it's hidden. Most people don't realise they have a belief system about this, as they've never questioned their food choices and have just accepted that this is how things have always been. But *of course* we all have a belief system:

---

[*] Advocates of the carnivore diet might believe they're a lion on the inside, but they don't have the wide oesophagus, large stomach capacity, or high-acidic stomach of true carnivores. Human biology is more closely related to herbivores, yet our strength of survival and adaptability is what allows us to be omnivores[77].

Chapter 3: Marketing and Myths

that's why we have different feelings about which animals are edible, which are gross, and which are pets—and why that differs from culture to culture.

It's difficult to pinpoint exactly when carnism was created. More likely, it simply evolved over time, stemming from the necessity of eating animals in our hunter-gatherer days. While it's now seen as normal, and accepted as a universal fact, it's still nothing more than the current mainstream ideology, which may one day shift. One example of mainstream ideologies shifting is during the Dark Ages, when everybody believed that the Earth was the centre of the universe, with all the planets and the sun revolving around our little rock, and Galileo was jailed for proving otherwise. It took over 100 years for his scientific paper to be removed from the Vatican's *Index* of banned publications, and more than 350 years for the church to admit he was right[78].

In another example, in 1846, the Hungarian doctor Ignaz Semmelweis was the first to demonstrate that handwashing prevents disease, but he was ridiculed and ostracised, and he died many decades before germ theory was proven[79]. No matter where the mainstream ideology originally came from, there have always been people or corporations who've benefited from maintaining the status quo, and it's no different with the ideology of carnism. Like the Vatican wanting to remain the authority on all things scripture, and the doctors who didn't want to be blamed for infecting their patients, the animal agriculture industries want to retain their profits.

A variety of factors are at play to keep an ideology alive. As mentioned in the start of this chapter, the main way a belief system continues to exist is to convince us that it's normal, natural, and necessary. Two of the ways in which carnism convinces us that it's normal to eat animals is through objectification and de-individualisation. For example, instead of seeing animals as sentient beings, we treat them as objects, products or things, and rather than individuals with unique lives and experiences, we group them together as 'livestock' or 'cattle'. Yet anyone who works closely with animals will confirm that they have personalities and preferences, no different from our pets that we cuddle, play with, and let lick our faces. Even small family farmers I've spoken with know all their animals by name and can identify their unique quirks. It doesn't help that the handful of species we've chosen to eat are selectively bred to be genetically similar, so we see even less variation than there naturally would be.

A third aspect of how we've normalised this belief system is that it's baked into our identity. To start with, there's the religious dogma that God gave us dominion over the animals, and so therefore it's our right to eat them. Even if we're not religious, we've all seen the hypothetically invented 'food chain', which (of course) places humans at the top. This is nothing more than ego: the reality is more like a food 'web', based on a circular ecosystem in which everything is connected and impacts each other. We eat both plants and animals, and of course we know that animals could kill *us*, as can certain plants and even microorganisms (if we don't conquer them first with hand sanitiser).

And finally, the most subtle way it's baked into our identity—and I believe this will be the most challenging to shift on a global scale—is the link between masculinity and eating meat: not only is it normal, but it's desirable, and you're

Chapter 3: Marketing and Myths

not a 'real man' if you don't eat meat. Most likely stemming from the early 20th-century myth that strength comes from protein, and protein comes from animals, this idea that eating (and killing) meat makes you a man is fuelled by advertisers and fast-food chains[80]. Eating meat is supposed to be manly, and studies have demonstrated that men will eat meat when they feel that their masculinity is threatened[81]. This is what makes it hard for men to choose plant-based options when they're out with other men, even if they want to, for fear of being labelled a 'sissy'[82,83]. However, the real definition of a man is one who provides for his community and protects the people around him. In the old days, men became providers by hunting, and protectors by being a warrior. Today, more and more men are tuning in to the idea that being vegan aligns with the masculine drive for providing and protecting: it means standing up for those who can't protect themselves, doing what's necessary to look after our planetary home, and keeping their loved ones safe from harm and exploitation. It's fantastic to know that today's men are appreciating that 'manning up' (I loathe that expression, but it serves a purpose here) means more than not showing pain when they scrape their shins (although they should be able to whenever they please!). It's about rising up for what they believe in and making change for the greater good, and I welcome this shift.

Somehow, as children, many of us instinctively knew that eating animals didn't feel right. Many vegetarians and vegans I've spoken with remember the questions they had in childhood, and they were met with a variety of responses. Some parents were supportive right away, but other parents tried to cajole and convince, and, even worse, threaten, in order to get their kids to eat meat. They were told horror stories about their bones falling apart, or about them ending up weak and pale. When kids have made the connection between the food on their plate and the animals it comes from, one of the myths they're often fed is, 'If we want to eat food, it has to come from animals.' Other friends I've spoken with remember being told that the animals lived happy lives and died naturally.

I don't believe that this comes from anything more sinister than the parents not knowing any different themselves. Many parents know how hard it is to get kids to eat anything at the best of times, so they'll say whatever they can to reassure them that what they're eating is part of a normal and healthy diet. There may also be a fear that their children will struggle if they reject the dominant narrative[84] (which can most certainly have negative consequences—and require therapy—later in life, but that's another book altogether).

This is the power of a mainstream ideology that's so pervasive that it's not questioned. It's easier to just go with the flow and accept the myth: everyone else is doing it, and therefore it must be 'normal'.

Animals Are Well-Cared For

One of the main reasons parents tell their kids that animals lived happy lives is because humans are instinctively opposed to suffering. On some level, parents know (and this is supported by studies[85]) that childhood cruelty to animals is a precursor of violence and aggression later in life, and they don't want their kids thinking that harming animals is acceptable[84]. The belief that animals are treated well is important in order to continue consumption. For us to be able to justify to ourselves

Chapter 3: Marketing and Myths

that eating animals is normal, we have to believe that animals are well-cared for, humanely, without suffering, and then the truth needs to be kept hidden so that we can convince ourselves it's not that bad. Our last chapter exposed the truth of what happens, and now we'll explore the ways in which the animal industry uses marketing and myths to convince us that animals are well-cared for.

The first step is the appropriation of rural, traditional, farming values: the myth of 'family farms'. When I hear 'family farm', I picture a sweet little cottage, a veggie garden and some fruit trees, green pastures with chickens running around, and maybe a couple of pigs and dogs too, with a cow out the back[*]. For the same reason, supermarkets have been creating false farm names for their meat and egg products[86] to conjure up images of green fields and happy animals. But just because a farm is 'family owned' doesn't mean it's not an intensive factory-style farm. The vast majority of farms around the world are still 'family owned', yet nearly every single chicken farm in the world is an intensive-style chicken barn. This is why the majority of Americans believe they're eating 'humane' meat, when only about 1% of their meat is *not* raised in an intensive factory farm system[87]—they can't all be right.

Corporations and intensive farming are taking over small traditional family farms and decimating rural communities[88], yet they promote themselves as family operations in an effort to win public trust. We have an automatic association of family farms as run by kind-hearted, salt-of-the-earth, honest, and

---

[*] '…and a veranda out the front…' Are any of my Aussie friends now singing the theme tune to "Burke's Backyard"?

hard-working people[89]. What may have started as a single-family farm has now turned into large corporations that give their family branding to all the smaller ones they buy out. An example of this is the Thomas Farms brand in Australia: they genuinely are 100% wholly owned by an Australian family, yet their corporation, Thomas Foods International, worth $3 billion*, acquires meat products from a range of suppliers worldwide and rebrands them under their family-friendly label. Their website has pictures of cattle and sheep grazing peacefully on open pastures, yet they also own some of the largest feedlots in Australia[90-92]. What they're doing is good business, but their market strength may be built on the general public's pre-conceived notion of what a family farm represents: a pervasive myth that stops most people from digging any deeper or questioning further.

Relying on pre-conceived ideas is the basis of 'humane-washing'. Similar to the idea that polluting companies will 'greenwash' their products to seem more environmentally friendly, the animal industry uses clever language to make it seem like some animals have a better quality of life. 'Free range' is one of the most ubiquitous, yet its definition is vague and misleading. For example, conventional broiler chickens are kept indoors in barns for their whole lives (which can be as little as 35 days), and 'free range' only means they need to have access to the outdoors for a part of the day. 'Outdoors' could be just a small concrete area with a tiny flap or 'pophole' to squeeze through after getting past the thousands of other chickens. In addition, free-range chickens are only obliged to

---

* That's a larger GDP than around 30 countries.

Chapter 3: Marketing and Myths

be given access to the outdoors once they are fully feathered, which is usually at 21 days. So let's just summarise that: the minimum standard free-range label can apply if the chickens can go outside to a concrete slab for a couple of hours a day during the last week or so of their lives[93,94] (*if* they can still walk by that stage and haven't collapsed under their inflated weight). Not quite the idyllic image of plump chickens pecking around in the green grass that's shown on the packaging. Worse still, these standards aren't independently monitored—it usually relies on the farm manager to confirm they adhere to the code, with occasional audits from the companies who make money from fees obtained in dishing out the free-range label. Does anyone else see anything wrong with this picture?

Chickens aren't the only example of humane-washing. With pigs, the term 'outdoor bred' means that they're *born* outdoors but then brought inside at four weeks to fatten up. 'Outdoor reared' doesn't mean pasture—it can be as basic as an indoor pen with an outside extension that has access to fresh air (think of a hotel room with a balcony, except you're living there with 20 others)[95]. Even in the 'free range' or 'free farmed' version of pork, it's only the mother breeding sows who are kept outdoors; the piglets are usually always raised indoors once they're weaned—and remember, the piglets are the ones we eat[96]. Beef can still be labelled as 'grass fed' even if the cows spend up to 100 days in a grain feedlot[97,98]. When asked why companies use these different labels when standards are so similar, the CEO of Red Tracker (a prominent UK welfare labelling company) said, 'The advantages are [that] some people are prepared to pay more money for it because they think it's better welfare.'[99] Because they *think* it's better welfare. Got it. It's similar to the way that many brands create a premium product (think: sports cars), with the expectation that the halo effect of this one outstanding product will subconsciously rub off on their other regular products.

It's up to us as the consumers to make change by voting with our wallets, because the organisations and charities we trust to look after this aren't always doing their best. The RSPCA (Royal Society for the Prevention of Cruelty to Animals), for example, is focused on the *mitigation* of animal cruelty, not prevention. In the West, its work is focused on *normalising* our treatment of animals, yet in Asia it's working hard to *eliminate* the dog meat trade. Why the double standards? Possibly, they risk losing consumer donations if they come out too hard against the mainstream ideology, and they certainly risk losing licensing fees if their standards are too strict for the farms that pay to be licensed. But could you imagine the RSPCC (Royal Society for the Prevention of Cruelty to Children) working alongside child traffickers to ensure the children they take as sex slaves are treated kindly, with a large enough bed and access to fresh air? While the standards of the RSPCA might be an improvement on conventional farming practices, they still allow many horrible procedures to take place such as debeaking, castration without anaesthesia, and killing babies. As Ed Winters says in *Vegan Propaganda*, 'Just because we can do something worse does not mean what we're doing is okay.'[100]

What it comes down to in the end is that 'humane' itself is a myth, because even if animals are well-cared for, they're still slaughtered in their youth. Why would we think it's better to take the life of a happy, playful puppy that's been cuddled

Chapter 3: Marketing and Myths

and fed well, compared to one that was caged and mistreated? Some say death is a blessing for animals like this, but there's no need for a 'blessing death' if we haven't bred them into existence in the first place. And finally, there's no humane way to take the life of someone who doesn't want to be killed.

#OnlyInAmerica

One of the first myths I had to overcome myself—and one that many non-vegans often use as justification for eating meat—is that of, 'Yeah, but that's America—it doesn't happen like that here.' Unfortunately, wherever 'here' may be, factory farming is happening.

Every year in Australia, we raise and slaughter five million pigs, eight million cows, 31 million sheep, and 635 million chickens[101]—but where are they? I know it's hard to picture what this many animals looks like, but even when driving through the most rural areas, how many cows have you seen at any one time? A couple of hundred? Maybe up to 1,000 if you can see really far. The sad truth is that around 50% of Australian beef ends up on feedlots[102], with 90% of our pigs and chickens[103,104] spending their lives in huge indoor barns.

The UK and New Zealand, countries both characterised by picturesque, green, rolling hills, haven't escaped the US-style factory farm system. It's been revealed that the UK has over 1,000 intensive-style mega-farms in operation around the country, despite politicians promising it would never happen there. Most are for chickens and pigs, but exact numbers for cattle or dairy feedlots are hard to come by, since DEFRA (Department for Environment, Food and Rural Affairs) doesn't require registration for industrial beef operations, and so no official records are held[105,106]. In NZ, Wakanui Beef (as part of ANZCO foods) has owned and operated the Five Star Beef Feedlot since 1991, the largest in NZ with a capacity of 20,000 cattle. Most of its grain-fed beef is exported, and around 5% goes to the domestic market[107,108]. In both the UK and NZ, around 95-98% of chickens and pigs come from factory-style indoor systems[109–112].

All around Europe, the same thing has been happening. Since 2005, European countries have lost over three million individual farms (more than a third of their total), yet the numbers of livestock have increased during the same time, demonstrating a drastic move to intensification, with fewer farms holding more animals. The change is driven predominantly by subsidies that benefit large operations over small ones. It's the typical 80/20 rule, with 80% of the money going to 20% of the farms—the largest ones[113].

One reason we may believe the worst is in the US is because they are consistently in the top-ten-producing countries for beef, chicken, pork, and dairy. Yet regions like Australia, NZ, China, South America, and Europe are also in these top-ten lists[114]. America leads the way with cattle in feedlots, but Canada and Australia are #2 and #3 in the world[115]. Another reason may be that the US media is more pervasive and so we hear about it more, but also that the nation's statistics are more easily obtained compared to other countries.

One organisation that's attempting to make the numbers clearers is the Animal Clock[116]. Featured front and centre on its homepage is a rolling clock, counting up the number of animals killed for food each year, and underneath are more statistics about each region's animal slaughter. They have a

Chapter 3: Marketing and Myths

page for the US, of course, but also for Australia, the UK, and Canada.

When we see horror stories about animal conditions, most of the footage comes from the US, so it's easy to assume that it's only America, or that it's only bad apples getting the publicity. But documentaries like *Dominion* (2018)[117] expose the conditions in Australia, and *Land of Hope and Glory* (2017)[118] show what happens in the UK. With the minimum standards of welfare so low, and the vast numbers of animals being raised in fewer and fewer operations (they can't really be called 'farms', can they?), the numbers just don't stack up. To quote Ed Winters again, 'There have surely been enough bad apples to suggest that the whole tree is rotten.'[100]

Every year, we eat ten times as many farmed animals as there are humans in the world: 80 billion land animals (plus trillions of fish)[7]. Most of them come from those large, concentrated animal feeding operations (CAFOs). With 99% of American[119], 95% of Australian[120], 73% of UK[121], and 72% of Europe's[122] animals coming from indoor or factory facilities, you're pretty much guaranteed to be eating factory farmed meat even if the label says something nice like 'free range'.

Out of Sight, Out of Mind

One of the foundational pillars that sustains this myth of normalcy is its invisibility. It's easy for us as consumers to believe the rosy images on the packaging and websites when most of us have never seen giant feedlots, chicken barns, or even slaughterhouses. And there's a reason for this: if we don't see it, we don't need to think about it, and an ideology that remains unquestioned remains in power.

Our countries raise and slaughter billions of animals every year, so why don't we see them grazing the land? The majority of intensive farming operations are housed in rural areas, hidden way off the main roads, with limited signage and unmarked trucks. It's not easy for the casual passer-by to know it's there. Official statistics from government agriculture departments are also very difficult to come by. Yet organisations like Farm Transparency in Australia[122] and Counterglow in the US[123] are dedicated to making it clearer, providing satellite-layer Google Maps to give a birds-eye view of the scale of these operations. Zooming in, feedlots are easy to see, as the animals are out in the open, but the chickens and pigs are still out of sight, housed in long, windowless sheds, often with 40,000 birds confined in one shed[124].

Activists around the world are doing well at exposing the true scale of the industry, but another way it remains hidden is through legislation. Laws have been created to protect the animal industry from whistleblowers and exposure, also known as 'ag-gag' laws. One example is the federal Animal Enterprise Terrorism Act 2006 in the US, specifically targeting animal rights activists who seek to expose its operations. These laws prohibit entering, filming, and releasing footage of commercial animal facilities[125]. Even if the footage captured exposes illegal activity, the investigator would still be punished for breaking the ag-gag law. The industry has also taken steps to prevent negative press that would damage its own brand, like when the Texas cattle industry sued Oprah Winfrey for saying that BSE (mad cow disease) scared her off eating burgers[126].

The court process is also used by the industry in an attempt to retain the idea of meat products as the dominant

Chapter 3: Marketing and Myths

and 'normal' types of food. Many plant-based brands are hauled through the courts to prevent them using 'traditional' names like sausages, burgers, meat, and milk. However, if we look at the etymology of the word 'meat', it comes from the Old English *mete,* simply meaning food that we eat as opposed to drink[127]. Meat that comes from animals was originally called *flesh-meat,* where vegetables were *grene-mete* and dairy products were grouped together as *white meat.* Milk coming from nuts is nothing new either, as almond milk has been a staple since medieval times[128]. As for being confusing? Have *you* ever been confused by coconut milk, peanut butter, hamburgers, fish fingers, hot dogs, fruit mince pies, or Easter eggs?[129] You're more likely to be tripped up by 'white meat', because it refers to pork (which is pink), the dark thigh meat of chicken, and even duck, which is scientifically classified as white but treated as red meat in the kitchen! In fact, studies show that consumers are more confused when plant-based products are *not* allowed to use familiar words to explain how they're intended to be consumed[130].

Euphemisms are another way that get us to not think about what's really happening. At slaughter time, *livestock* are *harvested* and sent for *processing.* We eat *beef* (not cow), *pork* (not piglets), and *veal* (instead of 'baby male calf that came from a dairy farm and won't produce milk, so this was a more profitable option than bonking it on the head'). In 1922, Texas goat raisers collaborated to rename goat meat *chevon* to make it sound more appealing. Chickens have their beaks sliced off under the luxurious-sounding term *beak conditioning,* and while they're shackled upside down on the line being bled to death, this is simply a peaceful *exsanguination.* Not the kind of relaxing spa day I'd usually sign up for.

Whether it's corporations being intentionally misleading, or simply not correcting the stories we already tell ourselves, the carnism myth has succeeded in remaining invisible and unquestioned. When the truth is kept out of sight, it's easier to remain blissfully ignorant. When we believe that eating animals is normal, and it's 'not that bad anyway', the animal industry retains its position as the dominant narrative.

Pushing the Dominant Narrative

Animal agriculture has an agenda, and their aim is to convince us that they're not that bad. Not only in regards to animal welfare and the health effects of consuming large quantities of meat and dairy, but in the climate space as well. The meat industry has been using the same tactics as Big Oil and Tobacco to influence governments, confuse the public, and keep us addicted to their products[131]. In the book *Climate Change Denial and Public Relations*[132], the chapter entitled 'Cowgate' explores the lengths that these corporations go to the twist the truth.

As recently as 2022, the US agribusiness sector spent $125 million on political lobbying, which was even more than oil and gas ($91 million[133]). Over 500 individual corporations financially contribute to lobbying activities, but a report exploring the contributions from only the ten largest animal agriculture companies found that these ten have collectively spent approximately $200 million on lobbying and political campaigns over the past 20 years[134,135]. The purpose of spending this money is to influence lawmaking in their favour, block regulations that would harm their bottom line, and sway

Chapter 3: Marketing and Myths

public sentiment.

Worryingly, it was also found that all of these companies had either directly or indirectly financially contributed to the climate change counter movement (CCCM), which appears to be set up to fund and disseminate misleading information about the climate crisis[136,137]. Tactics of this movement—used also by the tobacco and fossil fuel industries—include denial of responsibility, downplaying any harm being caused, publicly attacking scientific research, funding their own counter-research, under-reporting emissions, and failing to account for downstream impacts of their actions (such as off-farm emissions). All of this seeks to neutralize the conversation in order to keep the true scale hidden. It's not only scary, it's short-sighted and irresponsible.

The way I see it, if vegans are wrong about this, then the worst-case outcome is that we may have gone through some struggles to change our habits and livelihoods in the process of eating more plants and stopping animal suffering. Challenge is character-building, right? But if the animal industry is wrong about their arguments (being that climate change is *not* man-made and their industry is *not* damaging it), and we blindly keep going like nothing needs to change, then the worst-case scenario is our planet heating up, our atmosphere disappearing, and Earth becoming incompatible with human life. *Incompatible with human life*. I don't know about you, but I'd rather have a planet to live on than meat on my plate.

The industry invests a lot of money and effort to convince us it's not that bad, but a lot of that effort is simply reinforcing what we already want to believe. In part, I expect that most of us *want* to believe the story and are happy to accept face value of what the industry says. Before I knew the scale of this, I knew I couldn't have killed an animal myself, but it was okay for it to happen (as long as I didn't see it, of course).

Animal agriculture—carnism—is currently the dominant narrative. Most people see animal products as a normal part of life. But we're coming up to a tipping point. The demand for plant-based food and for companies that treat our planet well is on the rise, and there's a big market now for more compassionate, sustainable, and ethical ways of doing business.

Myth 3: There's an ethical way to do it

The rise of free range and other 'humane' labels has been driven by consumer demand. Most people are kind, compassionate beings who don't want others to experience suffering. We're horrified by conditions inside factory farms, which is why companies have cottoned on to marketing their products as if they come from better conditions. But we're getting too savvy now to willingly accept the labels without digging deeper. This, along with the current focus on the environmental impact and sustainability of all consumer industries, has begun to drive a demand for truly ethical systems.

If we *do* still want to eat animals, is there an ethical way to do it? What about eating local and organic, or buying certified pasture-raised meats from regenerative farmers? Can't we go back to the old-fashioned, natural ways of farming that still give us the meat we want and are also better for the animals and the environment? Let's have a look at some of these concepts.

Chapter 3: Marketing and Myths

Local and Organic

Eating locally sourced food is often touted as a great way to make environmentally conscious choices. And it makes sense when you compare apples being driven around the corner to the local farmers' market versus avocados being flown halfway across the world, just so that we can have smashed avo on sourdough all year long. While food miles are important, they're not as impactful as you might have thought. According to the data, food transport makes up, on average, less than 10% of the item's total GHG emissions (see Figure 11 below)[138]. The majority of emissions—80% or more—come from how the food is produced and the impacts of land use change (such as deforestation). When it comes to animals, food transport for things like beef account for less than 1% of the total emissions across its supply chain, so eating local beef might be good from an ethical standpoint if you know the farmer and their practices, but it's definitely not going to be helping the environment. Kilo for kilo, carbon emissions from most plants are 10 to 50 times lower than animal products. We already know that going vegan can halve the CO_2 emissions compared to meat eaters[139], but going vegan for only one day a week has the same impact as an entire standard Western diet with zero food miles[140]. Therefore, the best way to reduce emissions from food is not where the food comes from, but what the food is.

Organic is another buzzword that sounds great but doesn't achieve much when it comes to animal food. A 2020 study published in *Nature*[141] comparing conventional and organic farming practices found that the benefits achieved by organic animal farming (such as less on-site emissions and greater CO_2 sequestration in their land) are actually counterbalanced or even reversed by the organic process itself. This is due to organically raised animals requiring more space on the land, taking longer to reach slaughter weight (which means that they're consuming more feed, more water, and having more time to emit methane), and being smaller overall (therefore a lower productive output at the end, so you need more cows to achieve the same calories).

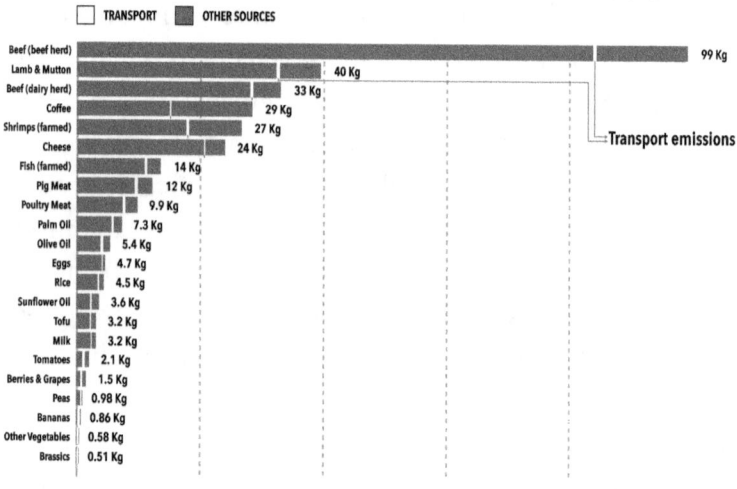

Figure 11: GHG Emissions by Food Type (Note the barely noticeable transport portion)

Organic feed for animals is also a contributor to more GHG emissions, as organic crops use less potent fertiliser, resulting in lower yields, and needing more land clearing and longer growing cycles to provide the same quantity of feed[142]. Overall, when comparing animal products to plants, the lowest impact animal foods still contribute much more damage than the highest impact plant foods.

I'm not saying that local or organic food means nothing, because once we're comparing plant products to one another, food miles and organic processing can make a *big* difference, but there's no point worrying about it now if we're still eating animals.

Sustainable Seas

The idea of sustainability is hugely important for the future of our planet and all life on it. Some of my favourite books to read are stories from ice-age fiction (anyone else love the *Clan of the Cave Bear* series?), and I notice how hunter-gatherers in these tales always know how to look after the land. They never pick the entire plant, ensuring that they leave some roots to grow back next season. It's the same with our seas: the idea is to only take what we need and leave enough so that the population continues to reproduce. That's why there are size and quantity limits on personal catches. However, these size limits and the actions of individual fishing are literally a drop in the ocean compared to the massive impact the commercial fishing industry has on our sea life. Sadly, more than 33% of the world's fisheries are currently 'overfished', with another 60% at maximum exploitation[143]. Since the 1950s, we've depleted our worldwide fisheries stock by 90%[144]. If we run out of fish, the ocean runs out of oxygen and humans run out of air to breathe.

And sustainability means more than just replenishing

stocks for next year: it's also about not harming the general ecosystem and ensuring that everything stays stable. Documentaries like *Seaspiracy*[43] have shed light on the issue of huge trawling nets that not only capture millions of whales, dolphins, seahorses, turtles, and other marine life as bycatch (which then mostly die), but they're also dredging up our ocean floor, releasing carbon 20 times faster than the deforestation in the Amazon[161].

So, of course, when we look to purchase seafood, we want to know that it comes from sustainable systems. When we eat tuna, we want to know that no dolphins have died in the process. Organisations like Marine Stewardship Council (MSC)[145] are supposed to certify and label sustainable fishing practices, providing consumer confidence in purchasing seafood. However, there's been some controversy over the potential 'greenwashing' use of their 'sustainable' blue tick. It's been claimed that they award the label to many fisheries 'with conditions', meaning that they're not yet sustainable and often have several years to make the necessary changes[146]. MSC has even certified some companies that use dredging methods and pose a risk to endangered species through bycatch[147,148], including tuna brands. That's right—'dolphin-free tuna' is not actually guaranteed to be dolphin-free. MSC also has an ethical conflict of interest since it exists not only to protect the seas—it was set up to protect fisheries themselves, and most of its money comes from fisheries paying to be certified.

If you're concerned about the oceans but still want to eat fish, the Marine Conservation Society has a website (mcsuk.org) that rates farmed and wild-caught fish of all species from all around the world[149]. It takes into account fish feed, habitat damage, bycatch, and fish welfare, among other factors, when giving its rating and is updated annually. However, unless you have the time and resources to find out exactly where your fish has come from in each meal, for most of us in the Western world, the best thing we can do for the sustainability of the oceans—and the livelihoods of island nations who *do* depend on fish for survival—is just not to eat seafood at all.

Regenerative Farming

In my 20s, I started to think more carefully about what I was putting into my body and how to be the healthiest I could be, and I think we all get to that stage at some point, don't we? During this time, I began eating more whole foods and adopted the Paleo diet. For Paleo diets, grass-fed beef is very important, mostly due to health reasons, as cattle in feedlots eat grains that aren't natural to them and don't get exercise, so they aren't lean enough.

During this time, I quickly learned that 'grass-fed' could also be misleading. Most cattle are raised on pasture to start with before being sent to the feedlot, so technically they can still be labelled grass-fed even if they're just finished on grains[150]. Afterall, they *did* eat some grass at some point. So, I looked for certified 'pasture raised' or '100% grass fed', as these labels ensured that the animals had spent their whole lives on pasture, eating and moving as naturally as possible. And when I went vegan, I still thought that pasture-raised was the best way to raise cattle for those who wanted to continue eating meat.

Raising cattle on green fields, as naturally as possible, is one form of regenerative agriculture, which is a holistic way of working in harmony with the land. Another is silvopasture, in which forest and grazing cows are managed together. With regenerative farming, the main focus is on soil health and involves rotating fields, planting cover crops, and no tilling, which not only improves soil biodiversity and water conservation, but can also increase carbon sequestration[151]. It sounds like a win-win, and there are certainly excellent examples of farms doing this well[152], but research has shown that these systems aren't the panacea solution they claim to be.

There are mixed outcomes associated with raising grass-fed cows in a regenerative system. On the plus side, not only is it better welfare for the animals, but eating their natural diet leads to better quality food for us, as it's usually free from GMOs and antibiotics. Undoubtedly, pastures and grasslands sequester much more carbon in the soil compared to dry feedlots. However, many of the studies evaluating these systems demonstrate that while they're certainly an *improvement* over conventional farming, the maximum offset potential is limited to only 20-60% of emissions from the cattle themselves, so the system is still negatively impacting climate change[153,154].

To start with, cows produce more methane when eating grass compared to eating grains, and since they're taking longer to reach slaughter weight, they live longer and emit more methane over their lifetime[87]. Living longer means that they also require more water during their time. In addition, studies have found that while soils can be a fast carbon sink, they may reach carbon equilibrium within only a few decades[155] compared to trees that can continue storing carbon for centuries[156]. And then there's the issue of all this extra land we'd need to accommodate all the extra space for grazing.

Chapter 3: Marketing and Myths

Let's assume that everyone in the US woke up tomorrow and decided that they'd only eat pure grass-fed beef, and that cattle production was able to change to meet their demands. Remember, 99% of meat in the US comes from feedlots or CAFOs. If all current beef production in the US converted to pure grass-fed, we'd need 2.5 billion acres of land[157]. To clarify, this is *more* than the total landmass of the US (2.3 billion acres), which includes all mountains, deserts, cities, and other land unsuitable for cultivation, leaving no land for any other agriculture, let alone space to build a Lone Star with parking for your environmentally friendly Tesla.

In reality, using all the current available agricultural land (without knocking down more forests or steakhouses), the US would only be able to produce 27% of the demand—meaning that we're all going to have to reduce demand for beef by 73% to make this sustainable, and then not eat any other types of food because cows have taken up all the arable land[158]. Even if we try to buy exclusively holistic grass-fed or regenerative beef *now*, it currently only makes up about 1% of the supply, so we can't all have it—and eating meat from other forms in the meantime is only going to continue fuelling the demand for factory farms.

So while regenerative farming and grass-fed beef is *better* than what we've currently got, in terms of welfare, biodiversity, and nutrition, it's not going to be a solution in the long run without also reducing our demand for meat in general[159]. It comes down to simple mathematics: there's just not enough land on the planet. Maybe back when we had 100,000 people in the world, sure—that was our way of life. We thanked the animal spirit for the contribution of the animal's existence, and we used the whole of the animal to clothe ourselves, build our shelters, and provide fat for lamps. But now there are over eight billion people who need food, and perhaps ten billion within just a few decades. And we've already seen that animals aren't efficient at converting energy into food. They take up 80% of land to provide 18% of our calories, and they eat around four times as many crops to produce the same amount of meat as if humans ate plants directly. Eating more plants and less animals is simply the economical choice for the sustainability of our planet.

The Beautiful Myth

It really is a beautiful dream to imagine the sun shining over rolling grasslands, clear streams of water, healthy animals, and a system that supports the biodiversity of life. But this dream is one of three myths coined by Melanie Joy as a 'neo-carnism': fantasies that perpetuate the myth of eating animals.

Compassionate carnism is what fuels the humane-washing and the desire to treat animals better so that we can feel good about killing them for food.

Bio-carnism is where we place animal foods as a central and essential part of diets, such as with keto or paleo.

And *eco-carnism* is what we've just spoken about—the idea that we can go back to the old ways of growing and killing our own food. Besides not being mathematically possible, there are many other things we did in the past that we wouldn't want to bring back into fashion today (cannibalism, child labour, or pooping in long-drop outhouses come to mind). These neo-carnisms are just another way we allow ourselves

Chapter 3: Marketing and Myths

to justify the myth so that we don't need to change our habits. Even if we wanted to, we still can't go back to the old ways of eating locally caught fish or growing our own food, because our human practices have poisoned our oceans and fucked up our soils. (Is that the first time I've dropped the f-bomb? My apologies—I just get riled up at this.)

When our human population exploded in 1700[160] (see Figure 12 below), we gave up any hope of returning to the 'old-fashioned' ways of hunting and gathering and living off the land. There are too many people on the planet for that. That's why factory farms took off in the first place, as they provided a cheap and convenient way to use the minimal amount of land for a greater output.

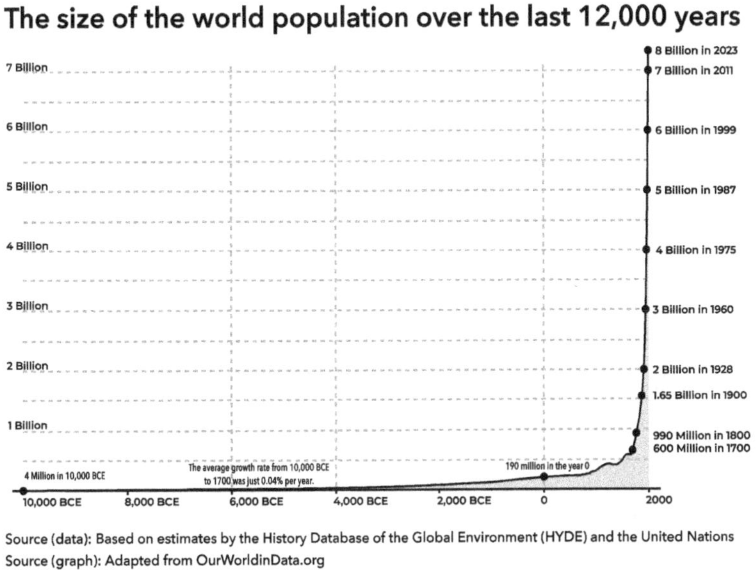

The size of the world population over the last 12,000 years

- 8 Billion in 2023
- 7 Billion in 2011
- 6 Billion in 1999
- 5 Billion in 1987
- 4 Billion in 1975
- 3 Billion in 1960
- 2 Billion in 1928
- 1.65 Billion in 1900
- 990 Million in 1800
- 600 Million in 1700
- 190 million in the year 0
- 4 Million in 10,000 BCE

The average growth rate from 10,000 BCE to 1700 was just 0.04% per year.

Source (data): Based on estimates by the History Database of the Global Environment (HYDE) and the United Nations
Source (graph): Adapted from OurWorldinData.org

Figure 12: Our World Population Was Minimal Until Around 1700, When it Multiplied 13 Times in Only 300 Years

It's that way with any myth—we only see the shiny marketing ad at first. We've now been exposed to the hidden and damaging effects behind the glossy brochure: the destruction of forests to clear land for feeding these animals, the horrors of their incarceration, and the pollution and toxic outputs. The corporations are trying desperately to hang on to the image of wholesome family farms in the idyllic countryside, but the writing is on the wall. If the United Nations—and a host of other international groups—is saying that the world needs to shift to a 90% plant-based diet if humans are going to survive, then it *needs* to happen. We *need* to get on board now before the change is thrust upon us. How we actually do that is what the rest of the book is going to explore.

Final Thoughts on Marketing and Myths

Out of the whole book, this Marketing and Myths section was the hardest to write. I've explained how a key tactic of marketing is to cherry pick sources and highlight one key feature. I'm unavoidably guilty of that myself, I guess—otherwise, each topic would be its own novel. I obviously couldn't put everything into this book that I've come across throughout my research, but the intent of this section was to share some of the things that, when I first heard them, made me feel not only scared and angry, but also disappointed in human race.

I hope the examples in this chapter highlight the absurdity of the status quo and have inspired you to question what you're being told and what you've always believed to be true. Importantly, I don't want you to feel bad about being fooled.

Chapter 3: Marketing and Myths

That's what the companies were trying to do—and they did a really good job. I also hope this section has inspired you to think more deeply about these topics rather than simply accepting what's presented at face level.

Here in Part 1, we've highlighted what's so wrong with the animal industry. The exploitation of animals is much worse than we've allowed ourselves to believe. Even if we know that animals need to be killed, the speed at which the industry operates means that slaughter is *never* humane and there is *no* kind way to take the life of an animal that doesn't want to die. The environmental impacts are scarily close to home, and the inefficiency of the system means that it's just not economically possible to feed our population based on our current demands and still keep our planet habitable. A plant-based diet is not the sole solution to climate change, but there is no solution without it. Marketing and myths have kept this hidden from us, pretending everything is fine, and obscuring the reality and seriousness of it. Corporations have adopted family farming values on their brochures, propelling the belief that what we're doing is normal, natural, and necessary. It's very sad that most people accept it as normal because, in truth, what we do to animals is far from natural, and the science is clear that it's simply not necessary.

If you're inspired to join me on this journey (and that was the point of writing this book all along), the following chapters are going to help you along the way. Honestly, even if you do nothing with this information except *think* about it, the seed has been planted, and maybe it will be someone else's book or a documentary that brings it to life. Whatever you choose, Part 3 will delve further into what to look for when researching, and you'll learn about the hierarchy of evidence so that you're armed with the tools to be able to evaluate what you're finding. Part 3 will also give you tangible, practical, and simple things you can do to support your transition to a plant-based way of living, in whatever way works for you.

But for now, Part 2 will make sure you're not getting caught up in perfection. As Simon Hill says, 'Don't let perfection be the enemy of the good'. We'll explore why a perfect vegan doesn't exist, and I'll reassure you that you can make a big difference in the world without being perfect at it.

Part 2

Letting Go of Perfection

A handful of perfect, purist vegans won't save the world. We need billions of people doing the best they can, changing their habits and reducing their demand on the animal industry, for us to have any chance at reversing the damage to our climate and building a world that's safe for everyone. I'm hoping that the first part of the book gave you the reasons and the evidence for why we need to be vegan, and now Part 2 will explain why it can be challenging for most of us. This section is all about releasing the restrictions on being perfect, understanding the psychological processes that undermine our attempts at change, and appreciating the foibles of being human. Overall, I want to reassure you that you *can* make a difference in the world—and encourage you to keep trying.

CHAPTER 4: There's No Such Thing as a Perfect Vegan

When I first learned about the horrors involved in animal farming and the logical plant-based solution to both environmental and personal health, I felt compelled to go vegan overnight, and a lot of others I spoke to feel the same. It's easy at first, but if we're not prepared for the long term, it can become harder once the initial buzz wears off, and many people may eventually give up on being vegan for a variety of reasons.

If you've experienced this, you're not alone. Here, I'll share with you some stories from others who've been in the same boat.

My friend Hanna and her partner were vegan athletes, and they even had a fully vegan wedding, but they went back to

The Imperfect Vegan

the mainstream diet (read: meat) after the birth of their child. Even though they both admit that they were healthier and stronger with plant-based foods, it was just quicker to throw a chicken in the oven than to prepare whole-foods meals from scratch. Plus, Hanna's mother-in-law cooked for them twice a week, and it was just easier to eat what they were given.

Connie was also a vegan athlete but due to stress-related health issues, she brought back chicken into her diet as a simple, convenient source of protein.

Another friend, Josh, was vegan for two years while working part-time, as he had a lot of time to make good quality food for himself and his two boys. But when he went back to full-time work, it was easier to eat on the fly, and so meat came back into his diet, partly due to socialising with workmates who ate meat.

Shea struggled with low iron even before going vegan, and she couldn't afford the cost of supplements, so under doctor's orders, she re-introduced small portions of red meat.

These decisions were absolutely the right ones for these individuals at the time, and you may have experienced similar situations. I'm far from perfect myself, and even popular animal rights authors like Jonathan Safran Foer (*Eating Animals* and *We Are the Weather*) admit to not being able to give up certain animal products or to eating burgers for comfort food.

However, it doesn't mean that these people aren't allowed in the 'vegan club'. Even though they're not doing vegan

Chapter 4: There's No Such Thing as a Perfect Vegan

perfectly as per the definition by PETA (who made *them* the boss anyway?), they may be making a huge difference to the world in many other ways. Many people have still massively reduced their meat and dairy intake, and only use it for the bare minimum of nutrients they require. Others are climate activists or, like JSF, authors who use their voice to help other people to change their ways, and there's nothing to say they won't be 'more vegan' again in the future. We should all be celebrated for the efforts we *do* make, not the things we're *not* doing. As JSF himself says, 'The important measurement is not the distance from unattainable perfection, but from unforgivable inaction.'[1] We're all doing the best we can, and to make a balanced choice instead of striving for unobtainable perfection isn't giving up or failing: it's being human.

There's no such thing as a perfect vegan: animal products are used so ubiquitously that they're in basically everything. And even when we try to be as plant-based as we can, we're not set up for success. There's a lot of pressure from society to maintain the status quo, and we also feel internal pressure from our own psychology. We envision unachievable standards that we hold ourselves and others to, and the way we're wired is geared towards fitting in. In the end, it's all about striking a balance between competing priorities and making choices that are right for us. Some days will be easier than others, some days we'll make mistakes, and other times we just won't care. Same as with parenting, sticking to a diet, and remembering to switch the lights off when you leave the room (as my husband is always chiding me for forgetting): it's not about being perfect every day—it's about consistency in the long run.

The Imperfect Vegan

Being vegan is not only about what food we eat, although that's the obvious place to start. When people go vegan, they often start by cutting out meat, dairy, and eggs, and food is the topic of most questions thrown at them from well-meaning family and friends. (*But where do you get your protein? What will I feed you for dinner? What do vegans even eat? What will become of you?!?*) Alongside the food is usually an understanding about not buying clothing made from animals like leather, silk, and wool. These are easy and common-sense choices to make.

However, the more we get into the vegan world, the more we learn about some of the sinister ways in which animal products are used and how they end up in products we'd never have considered. We try to be as conscious as possible by reading the labels of lollies* to make sure there's no carmine (squished red beetles), gelatine (boiled pig bones and cartilage) or edible shellac (bug juices. And also called 'confectioners glaze')[2], and we check cosmetics for animal testing and ingredients like lanolin, glycerine, squalene, and stearic acid (to name only a handful)[3]. But did you know that animal products are also in things like tyres, alcohol, plastic bags, and money?[4] I suspect I've just dropped a few bombs on you there.

Stearic acid, derived from animal fats and also found in cosmetics, is used in plastic and rubber processing, so not only is it a common ingredient in car tyres (although you can find vegan tyres, too), it's also used throughout the construction

---

* Also called sweets or candy, depending on where in the world you're from. But isn't 'lollies' more whimsical?

Chapter 4: There's No Such Thing as a Perfect Vegan

industry. It's pretty gross to think that the road you drive on and the house you live in may be made up of animal parts. Tallow, made from beef fat, is usually used in cooking, soap, and candles, but it's also an ingredient in the paper currency of many countries including the UK, Australia, Canada, and dozens of others[5]. When it comes to beer and wine, these 'good-time' beverages are often filtered with either isinglass (fish bladders), casein (from milk), or albumen (from eggs); and spirits—including pre-mixes—may contain animal-derived ingredients for flavouring[6]. A good time indeed. Alcohol producers aren't required to list all ingredients and filtering agents on their packaging, so it can be really difficult to tell just by looking at the label. Fortunately, companies like Barnivore[7] have created a website where you can search any brand of booze to see if it's vegan or not. Even white sugar is technically not vegan—the filtering process uses bone char. And, as I'm sure you're aware, insidious sugar is hidden in the most unnecessary places.

How Did We Come Up with This Shit?
Seriously, though—who decided to use ground-up and boiled-down pig hoofs for glue? My research reveals that there's a logical reason, actually. Our demand for animal food created a lot of leftover by-products: bits and pieces like bones, cartilage, tendons, hair, skin, blood, and basically anything that would otherwise go into the bin and create mountains of biological waste[8] (which is very bad for the environment). With our good intentions of wanting to use *all* of the animal, scientists were tasked with coming up with uses for these leftovers (the same way we try and figure out what can be made with ingredients in the fridge the day before the weekly food shop). And then, of course, good ol'

> marketing ensued to get manufacturers and the public to use their inventions[9]. The good news is: a) there's usually a plant-based alternative for everything, and b) when our demand for animal meat reduces, these spare products will become harder and harder to come by, and also more expensive due to limited supply, leading manufacturers to naturally move to plant-based alternatives for no other reason than they're cheaper. They're companies after all, and they're driven by profit.
>
> And, not to gross you out, but animal by-products also make it back into animal feed. That's right—we turn these poor, unsuspecting creatures into cannibals by feeding them their own waste products[10].

So, if we drive a car, spend cash, and enjoy a glass of wine after a long day at work, we may be unwittingly using animal products. And then, even after doing all we can do avoid them, if we're law-abiding citizens who pay taxes, our tax money is being used by the government to subsidise the meat and dairy industries on our behalf (thanks, folks!). Our money could also be being used by our bank or super* fund to invest in the animal industry. Since there's no way to be a perfect vegan, we can release the pressure we put on ourselves to get it right all the time.

This pressure is often put on other people as well, but we can't expect everyone around the world to adopt our Western vegan ideals. For most of us in Western countries, we're incredibly lucky to have access to food options and fresh produce, as well as information and the luxury of personal choice. A lot of countries don't have this. Around the world,

---

* For those not familiar with the Aussie lingo, 'super' means superannuation or pension, sort of similar to a 401(k).

Chapter 4: There's No Such Thing as a Perfect Vegan

there are many subsistence cultures who live in harmony with the animals they're growing or hunting for food, and they have a symbiotic relationship: without animals, they really wouldn't survive. It's privileged and entitled to think that we can enforce our Western ideals of veganism on cultures that would die without animals for food. In these cultures, we see what's been lost in our traditional farming values: the reverence for our animals and what they provide. The gratitude, the care, the compassion, the appreciation, and the understanding that we shouldn't take without need (like the tribes we examined in Chapter 2). On the other hand, several communities—like Buddhists, Hindus, and Orthodox Christians[11]—have been living the plant-based lifestyle for many centuries before the term 'vegan' was coined by the West in 1944.

Privilege is also assuming that others closer to home are in the same situation and have similar access to the same food, the same education, and have the same priorities in their lives. Many people simply aren't able to cut out animal products due to allergies or intolerances to some plant foods or lack of access to fresh vegetables, meaning that animals are a vital source of nutrients for them—and these intricacies can be different for everyone.

Social determinants of health also play a big part in choosing what to feed your family. The artificially low prices of some meats, milk, eggs, and animal-based junk food (thanks to government subsidies) keeps many low-income families stuck in a cycle of relying on what they can afford and what's convenient. People in poverty may not have the luxury of making the choices they want, and they may not have the mental bandwidth to care about the plight of animals when they're dealing with their own issues. But the more that people—with the ability to—demand plant-based foods, the more those products will become normalised and accessible for the rest of the world.

Part of my journey has been letting go of the expectations I have of other people. Just because I've done some research and made a decision doesn't mean that other people will follow suit. Especially those closest to me, like my husband and my family. I learned early on that putting pressure on others doesn't work in my favour. Instead, it actually gets their back up and makes them dig in even more to their position. I'd be far better off celebrating any small move they make, such as cooking a vegan meal for me when I visit or choosing the vegetarian pizza when we go for lunch. I'll use my real privilege to continue to drive demand for vegan products by ordering them when I'm eating out, and the more demand there is, the easier it will be for others to make the vegan choice, too.

One last reason that we can't be a perfect vegan is because we're not perfect in *any* area of our lives, so why would this one thing be any different? Think about it: Are you an ideal employee who's always on time, always giving 100%? Or do you check Facebook at work, browse your next holiday ideas from the office, or stay a little longer in the loo because you need to get to the next level in your game? Or as a parent, do you never raise your voice, never give in to junk food, or never stick the kids in front of the iPad for a bit of peace and quiet? We may have good intentions in all these areas, but the reality is that we're humans and we don't always do what we set out to do. There's nothing wrong with this. In fact, it's normal, and we'll explore that in the next chapters.

CHAPTER 5: Why It's So Hard

Going vegan overnight can feel like your whole life has been overhauled. Suddenly you need to think about food, clothing, and skincare. You spend hours in the supermarket googling ingredients. You end up having awkward—and often heated—conversations with bewildered family members. Not to mention dealing with the emotional toll from the shock of what you've learned, like where our food really comes from and the damage that's happening to our planet every minute. You feel alone, upset, overwhelmed, and disheartened. You struggle through the 'normal' way of life, in which animals are abused without thought. The yo-yo-ing from repulsion, indignation, and never wanting to spend your money on these corporations, to the craving for the comfort food you used to love. I know all about it, because I've been there.

Even though it can seem like an easy decision to go vegan,

it's very hard to maintain in our society: if it was easy, more people would be doing it. The fact is that society isn't set up for us to change, and going against the status quo is always going to be a challenge. This is also the reason why we need billions of people making a shift towards plant-based foods (without worrying about being perfect vegans) because it will swing the pendulum in the other direction, building momentum and making it more accessible and easier for everyone.

Having said that, it's so much easier now than it's ever been. From my own observations and from interviewing many vegans and vegetarians who have been living this way for decades, you can really see that there's so much support out there. There are many food options in mainstream supermarkets; lots of restaurants have healthy, balanced, plant-based meals on their menu (not just chips and side salad); and it's only a quick search on Meetup or Facebook to find local vegan groups. Many people say that food is generally the easiest part of being vegan once you understand the nutrients and how to eat whole foods (and there's lots of tips coming up for you in Part 3). Once you've got food sorted, the hardest thing for many is dealing with other people and with our own internal discomfort.

As we covered in Chapter 3, we live in a carnist society. Although we've already established that what we do to animals is far from *natural* and that it's not *necessary* to get our nutrients from them, it still is *normal* for the vast majority of people. When asked what's for dinner, the response is usually a type of meat, and if plants are even mentioned, they're generally a side dish. Going to the zoo or aquarium is a seen as wholesome family activity. Non-dairy milk has

Chapter 5: Why It's So Hard

to be specifically requested, otherwise cow milk is assumed. Vegans are the alternative, the minority. We're the ones who have to plan ahead to make sure we'll be catered for. We have to carefully check the labels, and politely explain our needs to the poor waiter who doesn't understand that vegan is not the same thing as gluten-free.

Just like the LGBT+ community who are constantly dealing with assumptions about being heterosexual (for example, women being asked, 'So what does your husband do?'), vegans are constantly dealing with assumptions that we eat 'normal' food. Recently at a work event, I politely declined the platter of chicken sliders with a 'No, thanks', and the waiter, presumably assuming I said no due to its unhealthiness, enthusiastically chirped, 'Go on, you deserve it!' Only when I explained, 'I'm vegan' did he stop pushing.

It's really exciting to see some restaurants flipping the switch on this, like Netherworld in Brisbane that serves plant-based food by default—you have to specifically request the 'carne option' if you want meat[1]. One day, I'd love to see supermarkets with a specific 'animal products' section—how absolutely phenomenal would it be to shop easily, knowing that whatever we pick up will be cruelty-free!

Even though it can be tough to navigate the food landscape, it's manageable. One of the toughest things for many vegans I've spoken with is dealing with family and friends. There's the horror stories of being disowned, threatened, or forced to eat meat, but there's also the more subtle reactions, like a distance opening up and having no idea how to bridge it. Even when parents or partners are supportive, it can feel like you're living in different worlds. When I spoke to a vegan friend, Tom, he told me that he comes from a family of farmers and that it took them a while to get used to his veganism. Nowadays, they always have a vegan meal for him, and they'll also buy vegan wine for them all to drink, but they just don't want to hear about it. It's really sad to think that he can't share some of his most personal values with his family.

Well-meaning family and friends will often question our decisions, and not always from a place of care. These questions are usually unexamined regurgitations of society's rhetoric: the myths they've been led to believe, like worries about protein, iron, or B12. Part of it may be concern for us, but they're also confronted by having their beliefs challenged, and the simple act of being vegan around someone who eats meat is already a challenge to the meat eater. Parents, especially, may try to convince their vegetarian children to continue eating meat because they may feel the child's food choices are an indictment of their parenting style—no matter how old the child is at this point!

Even without family and friends saying anything, we vegans feel a certain pressure whenever food is a topic, which is quite often in our cultures, as most of our events revolve around food. Jonathan Safran Foer calls this 'table fellowship', and it refers to the customs and traditions of how food brings people closer together. Think of rituals you have around Thanksgiving dinner, Australia Day BBQ, birthdays, Christmas, and other special occasions. They usually involve cooking, eating out, or sharing special recipes, and there's an unspoken pressure to uphold tradition, because anything else puts a strain on the relationship.

In my family, Mum has a recipe for Christmas Sherry Balls that was passed to her by her mother, and every year since

Chapter 5: Why It's So Hard

we were kids, my sister and I would make them with Mum. Now that my sister has kids too, there's three generations making them together. However, last year was the first time I attended Christmas as a vegan, and I was nervous about suggesting that we make a vegan version of the Sherry Balls. It's totally possible, I even tested them out at home first (purely for research purposes, of course). But the Sherry Balls are more than just a recipe with ingredients—they carry down a tradition, and tampering with that tradition could possibly lose its meaning, especially since my grandmother is no longer with us. In the end, although they all agreed that my vegan version tasted delicious and basically the same, they opted to make their traditional style while I made the vegan one separately. It's not the end of the world, of course, but it does feel like a separation between us, and knowing that I caused it could have been enough pressure to forego being vegan, simply for the desire to uphold that tradition.

Internal pressure like this comes from millions of years of our evolution as a species, and it's hardwired into our DNA. Of *course* it's not easy to overcome, and it feels painful when we try. Being vegan is a logical decision for me, but that doesn't make me a robot about it. I don't program my actions and then sit back and expect them to unfold as planned. We are who we are because of society. We are shaped by the people around us. Being human, there are processes inside my brain that are designed to protect me. Their purpose is to keep me safe, comfortable, and accepted by the tribe, but they're the very things working against me when I want to change and break free from the matrix.

All these psychological processes serve a function, and they generally come from our social instincts as a species who relied on cooperation and the tribe for survival. They're not *bad*, but it's important to understand them and how they control our feelings and behaviours. When we name them, we can begin to reduce their power and regain control of our own minds. We'll still *feel* the pull to be normal and fit in, but we'll be able to recognise the influencing factor and make a conscious decision rather than just go with the flow. We'll be able to greater understand ourselves, why we do what we do, and why it's so hard to have open conversations about this topic. Understanding these also means that we can have compassion, because we'll be able to understand what drives others in their own decision making and behaviours.

So, from the worlds of behavioural economics and neuroscience, let's explore some of the psychological mechanisms operating in our brains that make veganism such a fun challenge:

Cognitive Dissonance[2]
This is the big one: it's both the reason why we go vegan in the first place, and the reason others are so resistant to knowing about it. Cognitive dissonance is the uncomfortable feeling we get when our behaviour doesn't match our values—for example, that guilty feeling I get when sneaking a piece of cake while on a diet (guilty, but oh-so worth it sometimes). As humans who desire comfort, we'll do anything to get rid of that feeling, and the three options we have are:
1. Change the behaviour
2. Change the value
3. Justify the behaviour

Changing *values* is not something that can be done in the moment, if at all. Long periods of contemplation, research, and soul-searching might result in new values developing, but it's a slow, internal process. The logical option is to change my *behaviour* and not eat the cake because then I'm in line with my value of looking after my body. But we all know that cake is really delicious, so the most common outcome in this situation is to *justify* by telling myself, 'It's only a small piece' or 'I've been really good this week' or 'It's okay, there's carrot in it.'

When it comes to eating animals, most of us have cognitive dissonance because we care about animals and don't want them to suffer, and yet we *also* eat them. When this feeling becomes too strong to ignore, is when most people decide to stop eating animals. However, with a society set up to convince us that eating animals is normal, natural, and necessary, it's more convenient to believe the lies. Changing behaviour takes more effort, time, and often money compared to using an excuse to justify our current actions so that we don't need to change anything. Marketing about 'happy eggs' works because we *want* to believe in happy farm animals: it eases our conscience and allows us to continue. That's why the meat industry spends so much effort keeping the reality of farming and slaughter hidden from us, so that we can continue our behaviour with the justification, 'it's not that bad'. And it's why many people, like my sister, don't want to watch those documentaries, because they know the cognitive dissonance will become stronger than they can justify away.

The invisibility of carnism allows us to comfortably disconnect, deny, and avoid the things that are misaligned with our values. It can be hard work to dismantle the justifications we've told ourselves, and it's often easier to just continue pretending that we don't know. This is also the reason we feel so defensive when questioned by non-vegans: they question us because we've triggered their own dissonance, and they throw back at us all the excuses we've tried so hard to overcome.

Consensus[3]

Another term for consensus is 'social proof'—the belief that because everyone is doing it, it must be the right thing to do. It has an adaptive benefit to survival, especially in new situations. We're social creatures and we look to others for how to act. Does the old adage, 'When in Rome...' sound familiar? If everyone is running in one direction, our amygdala (the part of our brain that's always on alert for danger) kicks in without us even having to think, and it starts us moving in the same direction, hopefully away from danger. It's the same reason we defer to reviews on books and hotels, and why companies use testimonials to demonstrate that other people have already given their product a tick of approval.

You'll notice that food marketing heavily deploys this strategy. TV ads are filled with happy families around the table, warm and inviting and sharing a hot roast dinner, or friends joking and drinking beer around a BBQ with their kids playing happily in the background. It's unmistakable that the message is, 'Eating meat is normal, and this is what friends and family do when they have fun together.' This is one reason why animal industries invest so much in school marketing, building relationships with hospital cafeterias, and product placement in movies. If we see their food in places of trust (schools, hospitals, celebrities), then we must assume by association that it's a suitable (and healthy!) product. This clearly isn't always the case. In fact, it generally isn't.

Chapter 5: Why It's So Hard

Consensus works against us as a vegan, because when so many people are doing the opposite of what we want to do, it can cause us to continually question ourselves, and we may doubt that we're doing the right thing, especially when most people are doing something different.

Conformity[4]
Related closely to consensus is the desire to fit in. A really interesting and landmark experiment was conducted in the 1950s[5]. In a visual test, a group of participants had to state out loud which of three line options matched the length of the comparison line. Unbeknownst to the test subject in each group, all the other participants were planted as part of the experiment. The planted participants were instructed to intentionally give a wrong answer, even when it was obvious. The video showed the test subjects' increasing discomfort as the others gave the wrong answer, and, even though they knew it was wrong, 75% of them went along and gave the same answer as the others. That's three-quarters of test subjects who were influenced to conform, without even being told to. The results drastically dropped when participants were asked to privately write their answers instead of publicly stating them, demonstrating that clever people will go against their own judgement just to fit in, because it's more uncomfortable to be different than to be dishonest with yourself.

This desire to conform has strong evolutionary roots from when being different was literally a matter of life or death. In our cave-dwelling days, being ostracised from the clan meant being kicked out of the cave, and chances of survival on your own were minimal. Food marketing triggers this fear by showing us happy families and friends in the hope that we'll conform to their food choices to avoid being left out, and you can also recognise this conformity desire in public health campaigns to convince people to give up smoking. They often rely on the ostracism factor, using images of people alone, outside, and in the cold while they have a smoke, and through the window they can see their family and friends laughing and having fun without them.

While being different and standing out does drive some people, for most of us our need to fit in plays out heavily when we're with family and friends. We don't want to be the 'difficult' one at the BBQ or to appear different to our mates. My friend Tom, a plumber by trade, chooses to keep his veganism to himself, to avoid the taunts by others at work when they find out. This also plays a big part in why men choose the meat option when out with other men, because of the social pressure to conform to the norms of gender.

Lazy Brain[6]

It can often be easier to just go along with what everyone else is doing, and this is because we humans come with a lazy brain. Over millions of years in the harsh savannah, evolution has shaped us to conserve energy. Our brains seek the most efficient route and use the least resources to complete its tasks, which is important because our brains—despite weighing only 2% of our body—monopolise about 20% of our body's energy. This is why we have pattern recognition, stereotypes, and automatic reactions, all of which are lifesaving tools. If we weren't able to detect the stripes of a tiger hidden in the long grass, assume it was going to eat us, and react quickly to defend ourselves, we wouldn't have survived to pass on our genes. When we weren't hunting and gathering for survival, we conserved energy by not venturing out of the cave.

Today, that means that we literally judge books by their covers, treat people differently based on assumptions, and are more couch potato than Captain Planet. We assume that what others are doing must be correct (consensus) and go with the flow rather than think for ourselves (conformity). Our brains and bodies prefer to take the easy route, which means that it requires a constant draw of energy to make conscious and moral decisions in a world where the default is against us. This is one reason I'm so passionate about building a world that's plant-based by default—so that it's easier for everyone.

Confirmation Bias[7]
Related to our lazy brains, we have a built-in tendency to seek out information that confirms our existing beliefs and to ignore or discredit information that conflicts it (we've already learnt as a child what 'normal' food is, so why revisit it?). This is even how our social media algorithms are wired—they fill our feed with stories and ads that relate to what we already like. The main reason for this psychological trait is to minimise our cognitive dissonance—we strive to either avoid being challenged or to confirm that we're right, which keeps us happy and comfortable. So even when we want to stretch our thinking and expand our research, we're more likely to be swayed by media and articles that affirm our existing beliefs. Confirmation bias is also why it's so hard to have an open discussion with someone on the other side, because we each only see and are exposed to things that confirm what we already believe.

An important strategy for vegans who like to talk about the topic with others (and hopefully plant seeds that will one day change their minds) is to be across both sides of the arguments. Just like there are no perfect vegans, veganism itself is not a perfect solution to the world's problems. It addresses a great many issues, of course, but it raises some other concerns and there are challenges to be navigated. It's valuable for a vegan to know this information and be ready to talk about it if they want to get into (and hold their own in) discussions with others. Just watch any interview between Piers Morgan and a vegan to see the worst of what we need to be prepared for*.

Illusory Truth Effect[8]
Studies have also shown that the more we see something, the more credible it becomes. Repetition breeds familiarity, and familiarity breeds trust, even if it's not true. In the absence of all other evidence, we find comfort and safety in what is familiar. When there's confusing information out there, we'll revert back to what we knew first. This is one of the reasons why meat and dairy industries will fund research: to create confusing and contradictory evidence, hoping that people will give up trying to figure it out and just revert back to what they were told in school (usually by these same industries too, as we learnt in Part 1).

A second way that this effect is manipulated is by having

---

* Ok, maybe there's worse things than being interviewed on TV by an antagonistic pr—I mean—personality, but I imagine it would be damn frustrating!

Chapter 5: Why It's So Hard

the media bombard us with advertising over and over. All we see is packaging, TV ads, and websites displaying plump chickens with 'free range' labelling and green fields, with very limited airtime given to the truth, so we believe the story because it's more accessible and repeated. On the flipside, we also need to be careful when coming across information that supports veganism, as it can fall prey to the same problems. Many articles I've come across will reference some 'commonly known' statistic without citing an original reference, and it turns out that they're just repeating what they've heard from the vegan echo chamber. We'll talk more in Part 3 about how to evaluate information and check for genuine credibility, which is especially important if you want to add your voice to this cause. You need to make sure that your facts are true.

Sunk Cost Fallacy[9]
Another psychological mechanism for conserving energy is the unhelpful desire to not waste energy we've previously spent. Have you heard of 'in for a penny, in for a pound'? It's kind of like the 'go big or go home' mentality, and it's the reason why we persist with something even when we know it's not working: because we've invested time and money into it. Like continuing to eat the whole large box of popcorn, even though I feel sick halfway through, just because I've paid for it. It doesn't only relate to having committed money to something—it could be having committed a belief and action to it. I found it hard to give up my business as a marketing coach because I'd told so many people that it was my thing. I'd invested time in education, created a whole brand and public profile around that image, and had received so many glowing

reviews. Once we've started with something, we feel like we may as well continue since we've invested our energy into it.

It's a fallacy, though, because continuing with something that's not working will only make things worse. As the Chinese proverb goes, 'The best time to plant a tree is 20 years ago. The second-best time is today.' It might feel like it's a waste to turn things around now, but leaving it longer won't make it any better or easier. There go our lazy brains again, always wanting the easy option.

For those who feel that their identity is tied to what they eat or to the diet of people in their lives, the sunk cost (be it effort, reputation, knowledge, time, or money) they've invested up to now can be a reason not to change at all. I imagine it would be the same for farmers who've spent their whole lives in the meat or dairy industry who now find their values at odds with what they do (massive cognitive dissonance), but because of how much they've invested in this way of life, they feel committed. Luckily, many find ways to break free, like the two main scientists in *Forks Over Knives* who both came from farming families[10]. And there's even organisations that've been set up to help guide and support animal farmers' transition to plant farming, such as Farm Transitions Australia[11], and Rancher Advocacy Program[12] in the US.

It can also be really tough for any vegans who had to reintroduce some kind of animal product to their diet, like Connie needing her chicken for protein or Shea with her iron levels, as they feel like they've invested their personality in being 'vegan'. If you believe it has to be 'all or nothing', you're more likely to make a risky decision (like resisting what your body needs) in order to maintain the identity you've committed to. A better option is to embrace the philosophy of being an 'imperfect vegan' and know that you're doing the best you can with what you've got.

Temptation Tank[13]
Sometimes we're taught that willpower is like a muscle: the more you use it, the stronger it gets. And of course, practice does make some situations easier. However, our willpower is more like a battery—it has a finite amount that gets depleted throughout the day, and once the charge is gone, we give in to temptation. Think about the times when you spend all day holding back outbursts to frustrating colleagues, then trying to navigate traffic without flying into road rage. You're exhausted when you get home, but you resist the urge to yell at the noisy kids or snap at your partner. At the end of all that effort, there's nothing left in the temptation tank to resist the chocolate cake before dinner or the slice of roast lamb that your meat-eating partner has so nicely cooked up for their meal.

In our carnist society, especially for those of us who still like the taste of meat but choose a plant-based lifestyle for environmental reasons, temptations are everywhere—bus-stop posters, smells from the neighbours' backyards, and ad breaks in Spotify asking, "Did somebody say KFC?" The best way to manage a depleted temptation tank is to ensure that we've prepared in advance: never leave the house without snacks, and make sure you've got food ready to go in the fridge. There's always a vegan microwave meal in my freezer, and I keep a stash of vegan chocolate in the cupboard for when I need a minute. To recharge our batteries and keep them topped up, we need to make sure we're getting enough sleep, engaging in mindfulness, and practicing self-compassion—all things that support you in all other areas of life, too.

Inner Critic[14]
My final example of how our psychology is wired to prevent us from changing is that little voice inside our heads that says we can't do it...that we're not good enough...that it'll never work. As a protective mechanism to keep us safe and comfortable, our inner critic isn't striving to help us achieve greatness and create new things: our inner critic's desire is to keep us safe and small. It would be totally happy if we spent our lives on the couch eating junk food, because even though we'll be unproductive and eventually die of heart disease, nothing can kill us in that very moment. It's the voice that perks up when you're stretching yourself, when you're about to give a presentation, when you're heading into a room full of new people...and it's the voice that tells us that we can't be vegan because we're not perfect. And while it can seem overwhelming at times and never goes away, this voice *can* be drowned out.

I choose to give more attention to my inner cheerleader. This is the little voice that cheers me on, tells me I've 'got this', congratulates my efforts, pats me on the back, and loves me when I fall. Everyone has an inner cheerleader—you may just need a little practice to hear their voice, because the critic has had so much airtime. But just like you're beginning to ignore the marketing and myths that the animal industry feeds us, you can begin to ignore the doubting, nit-picking, negative critic. Even as I'm writing this chapter, I'm hearing

Chapter 5: Why It's So Hard

my inner critic complain, 'This is really hard, I can't think of what to say', and straight away my cheerleader pipes up with, 'Yeah, but you *will* think of the right thing eventually, so just keep at it.' (My hope is that my cheerleader was right in this instance, but you'll be the judge of that!) Your cheerleader will be invaluable on your vegan journey, since the whole world is set up to keep you moving in the opposite direction and things can feel very lonely at times. This internal voice is needed to keep you invested in your beliefs and to reassure you that you're on the right path, even when it feels really hard.

When all these things above are working together, it's easy to see why so many people give up after attempting to switch to veganism, or why most people never bother trying in the first place. When we feel uncomfortable with our decisions (cognitive dissonance), it's so much easier to justify our behaviour than to change it. When all our friends and family are still eating meat and don't see anything wrong with it (consensus), we feel the pull to go along with what they're doing (conformity). With our human nature to take the shortcut and the easy option (lazy brain), it's a big effort to change our thinking away from what we were taught in school and by our parents about what 'normal' food is (confirmation bias). The meat and dairy corporations want us to go along with the dominant narrative too, which is why we're bombarded by the media—which is really marketing— because they know that repetition makes it true (illusory truth effect). We've already spent so many years—decades for some of us—living the 'normal' life, and we don't want to learn a new way of living (sunk cost fallacy). And then, at the end of the day when we give in to our cravings (temptation tank), that little voice inside (inner critic) pipes up with 'This is too hard. Let's have the rest of that leftover steak and a glass of milk and go to bed.'

If you resonate with any of this, know that you're not alone! I've struggled with these and so has pretty much every other vegan (and imperfect vegan) I've spoken with. This is human nature, and it's how we're wired, but we also have massive potential for growth and adaptation. It may seem like an insurmountable challenge, but every little thing you can do along this journey is helping to create a more positive world for everyone, so please keep going.

While it can be an easy decision to make overnight, and there's certainly a lot more options and support now than there ever has been, the daily practice of being vegan is not always so simple. In Part 3, we'll go into detail on the things we can do to support ourselves along the journey and overcome these internal pressures, such as connecting to your personal WHY. But first, in the next chapter, we'll explore why occasionally eating animal products once you've decided to become vegan doesn't mean that you've 'failed', and how you'll still make a difference in the world without being 'perfect'. (And being imperfect is much more interesting, anyway.)

CHAPTER 6: Being Human

Here's a reassuring thought: perfection doesn't exist. Even a sunset with its beautiful, ever-changing colours—how many photos have you taken to try to capture the 'perfect' one? Michael Jordan wasn't perfect at basketball—he missed more shots than he made[1]. And Mother Teresa wasn't a saint every day—she was known for her hard bargaining[2]. Just like in any area of life—work, parenting, being vegan—humans are *not* perfect. In fact, as one of my early life coaching teachers said, humans are 'walking contradictions'. That's normal, and it's okay!

This is the human condition: we can know that something's bad for us and still do it, anyway. We say we'll never give our kids iPads, but soon realise the devices make excellent babysitters. We know we should eat real food, but sometimes dinner consists of a bottle of wine and a bag of Doritos. I'd be lying if I said I've never eaten chocolate for breakfast, read my phone in bed, or ordered three margaritas at once because happy hour was about to end. (Please tell me that I'm not alone in this…)

It's also normal to change our minds. Do you still love the same celebrities you had plastered on your walls as a teenager? (Mine was Leonardo di Caprio, and I'm probably showing my age there.) Did you end up in the same career you studied for? Maybe you did, but most of us didn't. As a kid, I turned my nose up at pizza, Chinese food, and burgers. And although I wish I still felt like that now, those foods are *yum*.

We act against our beliefs all the time. I don't want animals to suffer, but I *will* squish a spider if it gets too close to me. Speeding on the road is dangerous, but sometimes I want to make the lights and I put my foot down. I believe sex is an important part of a healthy marriage, but on occasion, I've pretended to be asleep (and I *know* that I'm not alone on that one).

I share these examples to demonstrate that we're all human, even when it comes to something as important as being vegan. When it comes to our vegan choices, we don't need to try to be perfect all the time, because it's just not possible nor helpful for our own sanity. Sometimes at a buffet, I'll ask for a clean set of tongs for the toastie machine, one without congealed cow excretions stuck on it, and other times I'm like, 'Meh, I don't wanna be *that* person.' Sometimes I like to take a stand and hopefully start a conversation by saying no to things, like speaking up about wine that's not vegan or loudly refusing the free Lindt chocolate on Qantas flights (mad test of will!), and other times I can't be bothered. That doesn't make me a hypocrite. It makes me human.

Chapter 6: Being Human

When we have an unrealistic expectation of being perfect, it leads us to believe that we *must* be a hypocrite if we slip up or get it wrong even once, and that's not a very motivating feeling. Rather than hypocrisy or the desire to be perfect all the time, we should be focusing on consistency and sustainability in the long run. Instead, if we look at being vegan as something that's a way of life, a habit, a long-term process, then consistency over time matters far more than being perfect every day until you burn out. When it comes to diets, studies even show that 'cheat days' are beneficial in the long run[3]—they help you stick to it and make more improvement and growth over time. And they also help us from not punching holes in the walls or irritably snapping at anyone in our path when that pizza craving kicks in.

We need to look at veganism differently, not like it's 'all or nothing'. This black and white thinking isn't applied to other areas of life. We're not a dishonest cheat if we tell a lie once. We're not obligated to give all our money to charity just because we donate at Christmas time. If I only get 90% on an exam, I haven't failed the whole thing: I've actually got a High Distinction. Building a plant-based world is not about 'pass or fail'—it's about progress and intention and compassion. When it comes to vegan food choices, Simon Hill says, 'Practicing flexibility doesn't make you a failure—it's smart.' In fact, in Simon's book *The Proof is in the Plants*, he shares eight principles for maintaining a plant-based lifestyle, and the final one is 'Don't let perfection be the enemy of the good.' Trying to be perfect can have a negative impact on the overall success of whatever you're trying to do, and it may cause you to give up completely because it's too hard and unrealistic.

The Imperfect Vegan

One of the biggest challenges we'll deal with as humans is to let go of the pressure we put on ourselves to be perfect. Life isn't a jigsaw puzzle, in which all the pieces fit together without any gaps, double-ups, or jagged edges. Life is messy and imperfect, and there's not always one right decision. Being vegan is about constantly making choices and finding balance between competing priorities. The original philosophy of veganism is not allowing any exploitation of animals—*as far as is possible and practicable*[4]—but people also come into veganism for health or environmental reasons. There's very clear science that, overall, a plant-based diet is better for us and the planet, but individual choices aren't always so easy and obvious. The decision you make will be the best at the time, and it may change the next time. That's okay! There are also occasions when you can't be bothered figuring it out and so you just go with what's easier, or times when you're prioritising your mental health with a day on the couch and three serves of Uber Eats—and that's okay, too. It happens to the best of us. Knowing that there's no 'one perfect solution' means that you can have compassion for yourself in every choice you make.

I'll give you an example of one such choice I made recently. At a work conference, we'd finished our catered lunch and were heading back inside the room, and I saw that there were several leftover pieces of tuna sushi on the platter. Knowing they'd be thrown away soon, I considered whether I should eat some.

I weighed up the options in my mind:

Chapter 6: Being Human

Why I wouldn't touch them:
- ✗ I'm vegan, so I don't eat animals
- ✗ Fish have microplastics and toxins from our ocean waste
- ✗ Farmed fish are diseased and gross

On the other hand:
- ✓ Eating them would reduce food waste
- ✓ Leftovers don't cause any extra environmental harm or exploitation
- ✓ The vegan options I already ate didn't have good quality protein in them
- ✓ I used to like the taste of tuna sushi rolls

There were many other options besides eating them or walking past—I could have found another group to give them away to. I could take the platter into our room and encourage people to eat the leftovers. I could put them in the fridge and bring them later to a friend who would eat them.

Everyone will have their own opinion about what the right action to take is, and that's evidence that there's no 'one perfect solution' to any situation. It's only what's right for ourselves in that time, and whatever option we choose today might be different from a very similar situation another day, and that's fine. Humans are walking contradictions, and that's part of the fun of us. (Sometimes, I'm sure my husband would prefer otherwise.)

In the end, I made the decision that was right for me in the moment, and that's all you can ask of yourself: to make the choice that's right for *you*, but to make the choice with *intention*. Rather than blindly following taste, society, or what's 'normal', pause for a moment to weigh up as many factors as you can (that you know about) and think about your choices. If you make a different choice next time, that's fine. If you learn some new information that would've made previous choices different, okay—well, now you know for the future. It's not about being perfect, it's about being *intentional*.*

~

Letting go of perfection also means letting go of *others* being perfect. Everyone is on their own journey and comes to their own conclusions. And just like it's okay for me to change my mind and make balanced choices, it's also okay for them, too. If we hold people to the 'all or nothing' standard when it comes to being vegan, they're more likely to completely revert to the mainstream diet rather than continuing to do the best they can with small choices.

Companies can be human, too. There are so many small business brands that are joining the mission of creating a plant-based world, and these companies are run by humans who might make mistakes and need our support, not our condemnation. I'm thinking specifically of the brand Impossible, which makes plant-based meat products that look, taste, and bleed like meat from animals. It's fully plant-based, but if you've spent any time in vegan Facebook groups, you'll have heard the company being slammed for not being fully vegan[5,6].

Its mission is the same as mine—to create a world that's plant-based by default—and it contributes to this by creating

---

* You're likely curious about the choice I made, but sorry to disappoint. My decision isn't what's important here—the *thought process* is. The point is that there *is* no perfect decision and everyone is free to make their own choices.

products that replicate meat, providing something so similar in taste that meat eaters won't know the difference. And it works. The company's blind taste tests show that even the burliest of self-professed carnivores enjoy the taste[7–9]. But it's not only taste—with a very similar nutrient profile, including iron and protein, the production of Impossible meats also uses 87% less water, 96% less land, and produces 89% less GHG emissions and 92% less water pollution compared to the production of beef[10]. However, along its journey to a plant-based world, the company was faced with, dare I use the pun, an impossible decision.

Its unique meat-replicating ingredient—a plant-based heme product extracted from soy—had never been used this way before, so they had an expert scientific panel conduct rigorous testing to ensure the product was deemed GRAS (or 'generally recognised as safe', an FDA designation) for human consumption, and the panel unanimously agreed that it was[11]. While this is perfectly legal and acceptable for many food producers and local restaurants that would sell Impossible, most of the larger food brands, international producers, and supermarket chains needed full FDA approval before they'd sell the product. In order to achieve its mission of creating plant-based meat that the world could switch to, Impossible needed a global reach. But, unfortunately, the FDA's approval process requires testing on animals. Pat O. Brown, the founder and CEO at the time, wrote an open letter explaining the heart-wrenching decision to subject 188 laboratory rats to testing, followed by them being euthanised[12]. It was the minimum requirement, and it was a one-off procedure, never having to be repeated. I'm laying my cards on the table here, but as a vegan who wants to see a plant-based world, I support the company's decision.

With FDA approval, Impossible was able to launch into supermarkets, fast food chains, and mass-market distribution. Its global reach now inspires other plant-based meat companies to raise their standards and compete, which is good for us as consumers because we have more products to choose from. Having lots of products in the market normalises the idea of plant-based meats. Plus, future food brands that want to make use of this heme product can do so without having to go through animal testing. PETA made a big song and dance about Impossible not being vegan because of this one instance, but PETA also gives its stamp of approval to many cosmetics and skincare brands that have a vegan range, yet whose parent companies regularly test on animals and use animal products as ingredients[*]. However, we must remember that PETA is also run by humans (who are walking contradictions), and it's normal to expect that it has double standards and makes different decisions on different days, just like we do.

~

Many of us went into veganism because of compassion for the animals, and now we need to extend that compassion not only to others, but to ourselves as well. We're human: we make mistakes, we change our minds, and we're driven by

---

[*] I use Simple, a UK brand of skincare owned by Unilever. Most of the Simple range is vegan and has PETA's stamp, even though some Simple products still have beeswax in them (those ones don't have the stamp), and their parent company most certainly is not vegan. So, some double standards here.

Chapter 6: Being Human

internal forces that we often don't even detect. We'll either go through life beating up on ourselves for our tiny errors, or we can love ourselves and the journey we're on. We can focus on the good, on all the times that we've made the right choice and lived in accordance with our morals. We can keep making choices based on balance; we can recognise that there is no perfect solution; we can forgive ourselves for not knowing; and we can use our inner cheerleader to help us back up when we slip. We can even have compassion for not having compassion, remembering that it's a journey and it's going to take a lifetime. One person doesn't change the world by trying to be perfect and attempting to hold everyone else to the same unrealistic standards. But every one of us *will* change the world when we're all doing the best we can and supporting others along the same journey.

Final Thoughts on Part 2

In one study evaluating why people gave up their plant-based diets, nearly half stated that it was because they couldn't be 'perfect' at it[13]. If the goal wasn't perfection, and instead the goal was progress, intention, and consistency, maybe more people would be able to consider themselves vegan or plant-based. Deciding to be vegan is easy, but the everyday actions to live that decision can be challenging. Like all good things, we don't do it because it's easy, and we don't even do it because we like the challenge: we do it because it's *worthwhile*. The challenge and struggle of choosing morals over taste can be what defines us, and it's character-building. Like any challenge—such as sport, business, writing a book, quitting sugar, quitting smoking—it's never smooth sailing. There'll be plenty of ups and downs, failures, setbacks, small wins, and slow progress. The most important thing is consistency over time. Our ability to stick with it, come back to it, re-engage, and carry on is what will motivate us and inspire others.

If we all choose plant-based as often as we can, we'll make it easier for everyone in the world. Plant-based will become the default. It will become the new social norm. We just need to push the boulder until we get to our tipping point, and then the rest will fall into place.

~

I know there's going to be people reading this who don't agree with the idea of consistency and self-compassion instead of striving for perfection. They'll say that there's no choice for the animals, so why should *we* get to choose? Farmed animals don't get to have 'cheat days', and it's an insult that we can be so flippant about their suffering. These are the militant vegans, the purists, who won't eat at the same table where animals are served, who need separate utensils in the kitchen, and who'll call out anyone who makes one tiny mistake. And I get that. I've felt the same way, especially at the start of my exploration into veganism. I was angry at the factory farmers, the governments for letting it happen, the people who blindly supported the industry...I was angry at the whole damn system. But I learnt very quickly that me attacking everyone I came into contact with wasn't going to change anything.

However, with a lens of compassion, I can appreciate the

benefit of these strict vegans. I don't advocate for strictness myself, but I'm glad that *they* do, because they show us what's possible. They push the envelope, keep us honest, make us take notice, and never let us forget what we're fighting for. The true and original intent of veganism is animal justice, but to affect long-term change that actually breaks the system, we need to first make change sustainable within ourselves. It might mean taking longer to adapt fully, but once there's a majority, it'll become easier and easier for the whole cause. I'm okay with being an imperfect vegan, and I'm okay with purist vegans not being okay with me, and I'll continue to use my voice to influence and support the vast majority of people to change their habits. If you're okay with that plan, let's move on to Part 3 as we figure out what we can do to change the world in a way that works for us.

Part 3

What You Can Do

Now that you're ready to make a difference in the world, the following chapters will help you to do that. What follows are simply suggestions—they're not a prescription or a model that you *must* follow. You know what your body needs, you know your priorities, and you know how your relationships work. Only you can decide the best course of action. Take what works and leave the rest.

CHAPTER 7: We Need to Do Something

I'm about to kick off this chapter with a pretty bold statement, but if you've kept up with me so far, I think you'll agree that it's right on the money.

Considering all the points of impact—land use, water use, pollution, biodiversity loss, carbon emissions, animal cruelty, and human health—the animal agriculture industry is the most destructive for our planet.

This destruction is happening so fast that we can't sit back and wait for government policies to come into play, or for organisations to invent creative solutions for us. We need to get involved *now*.

As a planet, we need to drastically reduce our meat and dairy consumption in order to reverse climate change. Even though animal agriculture is not the only contributor to the problem, the science is clear: without addressing what we eat,

Chapter 7: We Need to Do Something

we won't make it. Simple and sad as that.

As JSF said in *We Are the Weather*, 'Intellectually accepting the truth ... won't save us.' It's one thing to know and to understand and to believe what's happening, and it's quite another thing to take action and make a contribution to the solution.

It may seem overwhelming, I know. How can one person change the world? Honestly, what I put on my plate really doesn't affect the world at all—but what *every* individual puts on their plate *does*. In our global ecosystem, individual choices affect the collective. Eating is a personal choice, but it's also *not* a personal choice. It's personal because only *we* can decide what we put on our plate, and we have to make the decision ourselves—no one can force us. But it's also *not* personal because our food choices *do* impact the rest of the world. Choosing a diet that considers water use, land use, carbon emissions, and habitat destruction has an impact on everyone else: We all live on this one planet.

A plant-based diet is the obvious choice, and it's supported by science. Chapter 1 laid out the evidence for plant-based diets and their overall sustainability compared to meat diets. And in Chapter 3, we learnt about the EAT-Lancet study with its aim to define the most suitable diet for a world of ten billion people by 2050, taking into account how we'd all live sustainably on our planet with the systems we've currently got. Even though other studies recommend plant-exclusive as the best diet for the climate, EAT-Lancet described a model that most people could achieve and stick to while still being beneficial for our planet. While its recommendation for an 88% plant-based diet still allows for 12% of our calories to come from meat, dairy, or eggs, this is still a significant reduction from the standard Western diet. It means that we're all going to have to adjust our palettes and get used to plants, because animal products will be harder to come by and more expensive due to their scarcity. The next few chapters will explore how we can transition to—and stick with—this new way of living.

To be clear, I'm not saying that diet alone is going to solve the issue. We do need government policies to change. We need better (and more honest) dietary guidelines. We need to stop allowing industry to influence our governments and science. Corporations need to be held to account for their off-farm actions. Pricing needs to reflect the true cost of meat, and not be propped up by subsidies. We need support for farmers who transition away from animals to plants. We need doctors to receive better nutritional training. We need food manufacturers to create delicious and wholesome plant-based products. Textiles, construction, cosmetics, and other industries need to move away from animal by-products and ban animal testing.

But all these things are big and slow, and they require a lot of people working collectively. And even still, they're driven by consumer demand. This world I've described above isn't some dystopian impossibility—this world is *within our reach*. Honestly. We just need more people to finally 'get it', and hopefully by this point in the book, everything's starting to click.

It's easy to tell ourselves that individual action is futile, so why even try? But the truth is that *because* individual action is so inconsequential, this is why *everyone* needs to try. There was a riddle I heard once about a house on fire,

Chapter 7: We Need to Do Something

and all the townspeople came to throw their buckets of water on the house. They were all working as hard as they could, but each splash of the bucket didn't do a thing. The change happened when they suddenly all came together, waited until everyone was ready, and threw their buckets all at the same time, successfully putting out the fire. Their individual splashes didn't help, but everyone working together at the same time saved the day. Little pockets of perfect vegans, no matter how hard they work at it, won't extinguish the fires of the animal industry that have long been ablaze. It's only when all the townspeople (that's us!) come together and make a collective effort at the *same time* that it'll make a difference.

You might recall that I've mentioned a few times Jonathan Safran Foer's fantastic book *We Are The Weather*[1]. Among other memorable and intriguing pieces of wisdom in it, he says the following when referring to the fact that one of the most infectious diseases the human race has ever seen was cured by a shared mission: 'Who cured polio? No one did. Everyone did.' Well, I'd like to exercise a little of my artistic license to borrow that sentiment for our shared mission here:

Who saved the world?
No one did.
Yeah, but who saved the world?
Everyone did.

Thank you—truly—for the inspiration, Jonathan. I kind of want to get this saying engraved on something and hang it on the wall—maybe near the kitchen to remind me of my mission when I see Phil pulling his steak out of the fridge.

The single most important way we can influence change, as individuals, is to decide what ends up on our plates. It's the easy action. It's something we do at least three times a day, every day. Individual action isn't letting governments and corporations off the hook. We buy it, so they make it. When we pick up some steak in the supermarket, that tells the supermarket to order more from the farmer, so the farmer continues to breed cattle. If meat was sitting unsold in the fridges, why would they continue to breed animals for slaughter if they weren't going to make money off them? How would they lobby the government if we didn't give them money by buying their products? Purchasing what they sell is giving them the green light to continue what they do—it's giving them our stamp of approval. We can't say, 'What you do is wrong!' and then continue to buy their products. Why would they change unless it affects their bottom line? For me personally, voting with my wallet is how I can change the world, but it took some time for me to get to this point.

My Vegan Transition Story

Although I have a couple of vegan friends (more now than before, of course), and have watched documentaries like *The Game Changers*[2], *Forks Over Knives*[3], and *What the Health*[4] from a health perspective, it just didn't click about the animals or the environment until I read Melanie Joy's book on the psychology of carnism, *Why We Love Dogs*[5]. I was outraged when learning what goes on, disappointed in myself for not knowing, and in disbelief that so much happens without us even realising.

Chapter 7: We Need to Do Something

As an Australian, though, I held onto the myth of 'only in America' until I watched *Dominion*[6] and then did some research on the *Farm Transparency*[7] website, both of which are Australian-based. After that, I was convinced, and I devoured everything I could on the topic. I watched *Cowspiracy*[8] and *Seaspiracy*[9] in the same night. I listened to Ed Winters' *Vegan Propaganda*[10] in one weekend; and Simon Hill's *Proof is in the Plants*[11] became my go-to reference for health and whole foods.

I felt power in not buying the products of this destructive industry, so that was my first action, and food is where I started. Because health was important to me, I worked with a dietitian for the first three months, got my bloods checked regularly, and tracked my food with the Chronometer app to ensure I was meeting nutrient requirements. Online, I discovered heaps of delicious-sounding recipes, and created lists of ones to try and places to eat out at.

I'm usually someone who loves variety, but all this actually made me feel overwhelmed. All these new tastes, different products to learn about, and cooking methods to get used to were too much. For me, my diet wasn't only about ensuring it included no animal products, but also trying to be as minimally processed as possible, without added sugar, and meeting all my nutritional requirements. In other words, a healthy, whole foods plant-based diet. On the one hand, it's easy to not eat animals, but it does take more preparation and planning to create a balanced diet without them.

Something that was really helpful for me at the start is that I wrote out a one-day meal plan and just ate the same meals for two weeks straight. To me, this wasn't restrictive: it was freedom. I didn't have to think about food—just make it. After a few weeks, I let inspiration take over and I started making some alterations, like changing the salad ingredients in my lunchtime wrap or experimenting with new types of canned beans. It was easy to do, and it got me into the habit of eating healthy, plant-based whole foods. Now I can easily throw together a buddha bowl or whip up a casserole and get inventive with toppings for my corn cakes. Ever had them with avocado, smashed chickpeas, a drizzle of lime juice, salt, and chilli flakes? Sublime.

I've got some really good routines and habits now, but even though it was an overnight *decision*, it certainly wasn't an overnight *change* for me. The first weekend after I'd decided, we went away with my cousin and his family for Easter to their holiday home. He'd already bought all the food, so I ate the same as everyone else, just less of the meat items. When we went to the pub, I chose vegetarian meals. I just took it super slowly and was really kind to myself. I also didn't want to tell my family straight away, because I didn't have all the information myself yet and didn't feel ready to talk about it and defend the whole movement.

I did find that some animal products were harder to switch away from than others. For example, my usual breakfast was granola and yoghurt, and, at that time, the only plant-based yoghurt that existed in the shops was coconut yoghurt, and that's more like a dessert than a health food. Therefore, I opted to stick with dairy yoghurt until a better option came out. Within a few months, Vitasoy released its new soy yoghurt, fortified with calcium. And since it also had a high serve of protein, that became my go-to.

I also didn't throw away any of my clothing or cosmetics,

Chapter 7: We Need to Do Something

and I admit that I kept buying my soon-to-be-replaced skincare that I'd been using for about a decade because I didn't want to risk my skin breaking out. In the end, something happened to my skin anyway (curses!), and since I needed to find a new skincare range, I only trialled fully vegan ones until I found a brand that I was happy with. I also admit that I bought leather shoes after I'd made the decision to be vegan. I had an ankle issue and needed orthotics, and it was very hard to find the right sort of supportive shoe that was also vegan leather. I feel guilty about knowingly contributing to the exploitation of animals in this way, but I share this to emphasise that being as vegan as you can be is about balance—and looking after your own health, too. My belief is that one day, when we've passed that tipping point and vegan products are the default, it will be harder to get 'real leather', and so people in the future won't have to struggle with these choices.

My story isn't unique. The transition to veganism for me may be longer or shorter than for others, and I may have struggled (and continue to struggle) with different challenges than you or people you know. Everyone has their own story, so here are some of the people I interviewed and their stories to demonstrate that there's no one way to do this.

Maddy lived in a remote farming town in northern Queensland, and while she'd been vegetarian since 11, this town was definitely not a place to go vegan. Her only options in restaurants were the standard 'chips and salad,' and, being a farming town, she didn't have much local support. So she waited until she moved back to Brisbane.

Knowing she wouldn't be successful long term if she was too strict, she allowed herself a year of transition, being kind to herself by partaking in the office birthday cake or choosing vegetarian at restaurants if there was no vegan option. All the while, she joined support groups, followed vegan influencers online, bought vegan cooking books, and explored restaurants and vegan markets.

The hardest things for her to give up were cheese (naturally), comfort foods like Red Rock Sweet Chili chips, and a very specific flavour of ice-cream from Goodberries in Canberra. While it started with food for her, she naturally learnt about other things too, like which companies were cruelty-free. While she didn't throw out existing products like perfumes, she never bought those brands again.

Clark was brought up a meat eater and never questioned his way of life. Only when he met his vegetarian partner 20 years ago did he decide to switch his diet solely for the relationship. While he's now conscious of animal products in items other than food, he told me that he didn't even connect with the cruelty aspect of it for years—it was purely health reasons. Clark's contribution to the movement is setting up his own Facebook group for family and friends and inspiring them to eat healthy, plant-based recipes.

James loved eating (he's definitely not alone there), and even set up a university club called 'The Gluttony Society'. He realised that eating meat made him feel awful, but he may not have made that connection if it wasn't for his sister. Burdened with a severe health issue, she switched to a plant-based diet

Chapter 7: We Need to Do Something

in January 2018, and by June that year, James had seen the benefits and made the change as well. (It also probably helped that his new love interest was a very strict vegan, too. The things we do for love…)

James is the sort of person who goes all in, so overnight he stopped cooking steak and sausages and learnt how to cook tofu. In fact, he spent two weeks eating nothing but tofu, experimenting with different ways to make it taste good. Oh—and Oreos, of course, which in his words are 'everybody's starting point'. For him, he knows that willpower is not his strong suit, so it helps that he's got his sister and partner who eat vegan too, and he actually loves the limited menu options in restaurants because it makes for an easy decision when choosing what to have.

He believes that if it's important to you, it's easier to stick to it. He makes an effort to visit animal sanctuaries, check products on vegan apps, and learn fun facts to gently educate people.

Jasmin's first attempt at being vegan lasted only a month. She was raised by vegetarian parents, so she already had a head start on not eating meat, but even still, she soon realised that veganism was hard without good planning and preparation. She mostly just cut out dairy and eggs, but she didn't do research to find out what to replace them with. Her partner at the time wasn't supportive, she didn't know any other vegan friends, and university was stressful. Understandably, she gave up at that point.

The second time was five years later, this time with a partner who also got invested, and the two of them have been committed since 2017. They both had different approaches—hers was to get on social media and connect with Facebook groups, download apps like Fussy Vegan, and do the research. His approach was to read all the packaging, google the ingredients, even find out where things are sourced from. As you can imagine, standing in the supermarket aisle balancing a pack of biscuits in one hand and phone open at Google in the other, their first time food shopping after making the switch took hours.

Her desire was also to be sustainable for the planet, so early on into their vegan lifestyle, they continued to use up what was in the pantry instead of wasting food, and just didn't buy anything new that wasn't vegan.

Tracey is someone who knew as a child that she had an affinity for animals. It always felt wrong to eat them, but no one told her that she could live without meat.

In the early 90s she travelled around Europe, living out of a car with a tight budget, and ate meat maybe three times that year (nothing like being broke to thrust you into a new way of living). She realised she was still healthy without eating animals and didn't miss it, so when she arrived back home in Australia, she simply announced she was vegetarian. This was in 1993 and well before the internet, so it wasn't easy to find others. Eventually, though, she found a local group in Canberra and was even part of their committee for ten years.

Around this time, now that the internet was accessible, she started hearing about 'vegans' and was horrified to learn the truth about eggs and dairy. She gave herself a month to try being vegan, during which she got educated and realised

Chapter 7: We Need to Do Something

there was no way she could go back, so she stayed vegan. That first week was hard—she was *very* hungry. But she quickly found balanced meals, started to enjoy coffee and tea with soy milk, and got her protein from legumes. Luckily, she loved to experiment in the kitchen, and she was happy to throw things together to find what she liked. She still wishes that there was good vegan cheese, although she'll never go back to dairy.

At first Tracey was a militant vegan, wanting to educate everyone on the cruelty of animal agriculture, but she saw that it puts people off, and now gets a better response when she remains calm and leads by example. Even still, over the years she's made the hard choice to move away from friends who didn't support or understand her. As one of the long-term vegans, she confirms that she's seen a lot of changes over the years, and that it's definitely happening faster now than ever before.

Tamsin came into the vegan world from first-hand experience of seeing what happens to animals. Working as a meat buyer for hotels and restaurants, it was her job to visit abattoirs, farms, and factories. Even though she grew up in the strong meat-eating culture of South Africa and knew that we had to kill animals to eat them, she slowly realised that she wasn't comfortable with what she was seeing.

From 2005, she stopped eating chickens after seeing how they were roughly handled, often boiled alive. At pig farms, she'd see beautiful outdoor pastures, with pigs who came up to her like dogs wanting to play, and she realised she couldn't eat them either. Going out on the fishing trawlers made her give up fish, too. Beef and lamb were the hardest to let go of, culturally speaking, but living rurally in Queensland and unable to get good quality meat, she eventually phased it out.

And then on 17 February 2020, she moved to Adelaide for a new job, and went vegan on the same day. Cheese was the hardest to give up, more for the habit of using it as a protein snack, but an online challenge by someone on Twitter committed her to giving it up for three months. Even though she misses it now, she says she'll never go back: the sights and smells of the factories have stuck with her.

Tamsin found that social pressure was the hardest to deal with: not having decent food options when eating out, sneering by others, and the fear of being 'difficult'. She even lost friends for telling them not to bring meat for dinner. As meat is such a big part of her South African culture, she didn't know many other vegans, but she found she had a vegan cousin who had a quiet way of activism that she wanted to emulate.

While she admires the loud activists, she acknowledges that it must be hard to keep it up. Her way of activism is to politely ask for vegan options (for example, plant-based milk in coffee shops) and walk out if they don't have any. She believes that demand will drive change.

Even once you've made the decision to be vegan, there are undoubtedly going to be moments in life when you can't be as vegan as you want to be. It might be a health reason, it might be social etiquette (do you refuse to eat what your mother-in-law cooks the first time you meet? Death wish!), or it might just be taking care of your own mental health so that you can continue on tomorrow. Many people I've spoken with believe in the imperfection of humanity, and that sustainability is the most important element for long-term change. If it's not

Chapter 7: We Need to Do Something

perfect but it's sustainable, then it's the best thing for you to do. If this is you right now, here are some examples to prove that you're not alone:

Alyse and Jacinta run a successful fitness company, and while they're both vegan for the health benefits of a plant-based diet, they don't advertise as a vegan business. In this way, they've found that they attract more people, which may change more minds in the long run as their clients learn the benefits of the plant-based diet through living by example. Fairly genius, if you ask me.

Ashleigh struggles with depression, a lingering eating disorder, and a few digestive issues, all of which make it hard for her to plan and prepare meals. While she's mostly plant-based, she says that vegan pre-made meals are out of her budget, so she occasionally eats seafood and eggs, as they're easy to prepare and don't trigger her digestive issues.

David and his wife are vegan, but their adult daughter isn't. When she eats with them, David will buy a small amount of meat for her since she's not a big eater, but usually there is still some leftover. As David was taught to never waste or throw out food, he often struggles with the choice of eating the leftover meat or throwing it into the bin where it will contribute to the climate crisis.

Arriel was vegan for two-and-a-half years, but when she fell pregnant, she craved chicken from Red Rooster (that was my favourite place too, so I know how she felt) and so she brought it back into her diet. Even though she's no longer vegan, she's kept many of the vegan habits she learnt during her time, and she regularly cooks vegan meals for her family.

Rachel is inspired to do good for the planet and her own body, but she's not ready to go fully vegan, so her commitment is to go meat-free for three days a week, and dairy-free for three days a week. She's already discovered delicious vegan meals like cauliflower tacos, and even her meat-eating partner likes them, too.

Louise is 66 years old and was convinced by her daughter to go vegan. It was difficult at first, but she got used to the food and now enjoys it. Unfortunately, her body didn't adapt as quickly, and she had to have B12 injections and iron infusions for a short time. She's about 90% vegan, only consuming small amounts of seafood. With an artificial heart valve, she does what she can to stay healthy within the limits of what her body allows. Amazing for a 66-year-old!

Hearing these stories, it's heartening to learn about so many people being as vegan as they can be. I love when someone realises that I'm vegan and then starts telling me how they used to be vegan or vegetarian or how they 'did Veganuary that one time'. I sense an element of guilt when they say it, though, because they probably feel that they 'should' be doing more, but I love to reassure them that they're doing the best they can, and I love to celebrate the things they *are* doing. Human behaviour 101: you get more of what you reward.

Think about it: if you're proud of the vegan meal you made for your friend, and she complains that it's nice but it's

Chapter 7: We Need to Do Something

not good enough because you should be eating vegan meals every day, are you going to be more or less inclined to bake her a vegan shepherd's pie again? That friend will now be forced to fend for themselves, I'm sure. But if your friend says, 'Holy hell, this is amazing—I love it!' and gobbles up two serves after posting a gushing photo on the 'Gram, aren't you going to get straight back online and look for the next recipe inspiration? Even if we're not vegan every day, or for every meal, or there are certain things we haven't been able to give up, at least we're doing *something*. Be proud of it.

I tend to not broadcast the ways in which I'm not perfect myself (who does? Some flaws are best taken to the grave), but in the interest of reassuring you that whatever you're doing is helpful, I thought I'd share the things I still feel guilty about. I did say way back at the beginning that I can't write a book without being transparent and authentic, so...

1. When my husband buys a pre-cooked chicken for himself, he doesn't eat the wings (he says they're too fattening), so I eat them. Mostly to avoid food waste, but also—I'll admit it—I still like the taste.

2. I host a monthly conference at work, which I organise catering for. As much as I'd love to order a fully plant-based menu, I still have to cater for my guests. So while my order does include animal products, I do my best to avoid red meat products and cheese platters as they're more environmentally damaging[*].

---

[*] I've tried ordering mostly plant-based, but there's so much more food waste, because they just go outside and buy their own lunch. I'd rather provide what people will eat and not have it wasted.

3. I mentioned this earlier: I sometimes accept the free Lindt chocolate they give out on Qantas flights, because I love chocolate. I know that's not really an excuse, but I do refuse their other non-vegan snacks, because I know they also have a stash of plant-based chocolate and coconut slices, which they'll get for me if I ask nicely. And I do. I'm a very polite person. And being polite means that I receive chocolate and coconut slices when I want them. Motivation for manners.

4. I haven't switched to a vegan sunblock yet, mostly for sensitive skin reasons, but I know I'd try harder to find a better brand if I needed to use it every day (which I don't).

5. The popcorn at my regular cinema is definitely vegan, and most salted popcorn at cinemas is, too. However, when I go to a different cinema, I no longer ask if it's vegan or not, because I'm going to eat it anyway*.

Some of these things you may resonate with. With others, you may be thinking, 'What? That's easy—why doesn't she just do XYZ?' That's totally normal, and remember, we all have different life experiences, priorities, and knowledge, and we're all doing the best we can. I know I can do better, but I also know I'm doing a *lot* to help the cause. And, as we've already established in Part 2, perfection is *not* the goal. If I beat myself up for every little thing I'm not doing well, I wouldn't have any energy left to find new ways of making vegan choices—or to write this book, which will hopefully inspire countless others to do a little extra. I wrote this book to

---

* Popcorn might just be my kryptonite.

Chapter 7: We Need to Do Something

reassure people that they're on the right path and that they're making a difference in the world no matter how big or small their contribution. And maybe even to reassure myself, too.

For those who want to make as much of a contribution as they can, the following chapters explore some of the strategies and mindsets that have worked for me and others as we transitioned to a plant-based way of life. It starts in Chapter 8 with getting educated to uncover the truth about what's going on and learning how to evaluate the information you're coming across. Is it genuine, unbiased, with good-quality sources and high up on the hierarchy of evidence? Not only so that you know for yourself, but so that you can feel confident in your explanations to others.

Chapter 9 is all about transitioning to being more plant-based in whatever way works for you, and will reassure you that you can start small, make little changes, and build sustainable habits over time. Connecting with support is the focus of Chapter 10—not only connecting with like-minded groups and communities, but also connecting with yourself and your own WHY, and we'll explore how to maintain what I call 'mixed-veg' relationships. Finally, in Chapter 11 we'll consider how you can be a lighthouse for the cause—and it's a reminder to let go of unobtainable standards for yourself and others in order to inspire greater change.

Above all, remember compassion, for you and everyone you encounter. We're humans and we're imperfect and that's perfectly okay. Everyone's on their own journey, and while you may be revved up now and eager to *do* something, remember to go as slow as you need, make sustainable choices that you can maintain, and do what works for *you*.

CHAPTER 8: Get Educated

It's common to devour information when we first become vegan. We hear a headline or one new statistic and then we're off down the rabbit hole. There's so much conflicting advice from both sides, like how red meat is potentially carcinogenic but is also needed for iron levels. It's also easy to get trapped by conspiracy stories and speculation, and due to our inherent confirmation bias, we run the risk of only getting deeper into our own way of thinking if we don't stop to evaluate what we're finding.

The internet is an incredible invention—it gives us access to resources at an unprecedented scale. Twenty years ago, we didn't have such easy ways to find like-minded communities, uncover reports on government spending, or watch so many free videos on the best way to press tofu. I certainly wouldn't have been able to write this book as easily. But the downside

Chapter 8: Get Educated

of free information is that anyone can publish for free, whether that be a professional career scientist with multiple degrees and peer-reviewed publications, or a blog by a guy in his underwear in his parents' basement with an opinion and a drinking habit. Keyword searches give the same weight to vastly different qualities of information.

As a vegan, you want a certain level of education on these topics—not only because it's important to know the truth, but also because it helps when talking with others. Whether you're hoping to convince them or simply trying to explain your own position, it's helpful to be ready with answers to their questions about protein, crop deaths, nutrition, the way animals are treated in your country, or what's really driving deforestation, and for that information to be credible and trustworthy. For me, I wanted to know for *sure*. Going vegan is a big decision, a huge change of life. If I was going to give up and reject what I'd been taught to believe for the first 35 years of my life, I needed to know that what I was replacing it with was true.

The most important skill when researching is the ability to evaluate evidence critically. Critically evaluating doesn't mean criticising: there's an important distinction. Think nit-picking mother-in-law versus a tenured university professor. Criticising is picking it apart and highlighting all the bad points; critical evaluation means checking carefully and looking at both positive and negative aspects while keeping a sceptical mind. When presented with any new information, it's important to remain objective: keep your own judgement to one side, be aware of your own biases and assumptions, and try not to go into it with pre-conceived ideas of what the outcome will be.

No matter the format—article, book, video, documentary, report, social media post, et cetera—there's certain criteria to look for when evaluating critically.

Criteria for Critical Evaluation

The Author

The main thing I want to know is: Who wrote this and what is their expertise? What qualifies them to be talking about this subject? Do they have formal qualifications, or work or lived experience in this field? What else have they published, whether related or not? I also want to know who they're writing for. Is the intended audience their own industry, the general public, people who care about nutrition, people who are already converted? And what do they want to achieve—are they trying to change minds; promote the dominant narrative; share facts; get funding? What do they have to gain by readers believing this? Do they have any conflict of interest, such as being funded by industry? Basically, is this science or is it marketing?

Sources

There are two main criteria to look at here. Firstly, what type of source is your piece? A *primary* source is an original experiment or study, and a *secondary* source is an analysis or interpretation of a primary source, often an opinion. An example of a primary source is a study about protein intake for bodybuilding, published by the researchers and usually in a respected journal; a secondary source would be an article

Chapter 8: Get Educated

on a health website that talks about the study and uses it to justify sales of their protein bars. Further in this chapter, I'll explain the hierarchy of evidence, as each type of primary source can be evaluated for its quality and reliability.

Second, where does the evidence come from? Has the author even referenced their sources with enough information so that you can look them up yourself, or are they just spouting 'facts' without any way for the reader to verify them? Are they relying on good-quality, primary sources? Here's a fun example: In doing my research about meat consumption in Australia, I came across an industry report from a government organisation called Safe Food Queensland[1]. They made a claim saying that 97% of Australian meat is grass-fed, which conflicted with reports I'd already found that say 51% of Australian cattle are in feedlots. Their reference for 97% linked me to a blog post by a restaurant called 'Meat & Wine Co'[2]. The blog post didn't link any source itself: it just made the claim without any backup. Not a good example of quality sources[*].

And to demonstrate that I'm trying my best not to be biased, here's an example from the vegan world. You may have heard that 90% of B12 supplements are given to animals. This is a common 'fact' that was originally mentioned in a news article[3] with no reference to back it up, and the vegan echo chamber has picked it up and repeated it in perpetuity. But no matter how deep I've scoured, I haven't found any official documents to back it up. I'd really love to find evidence of it, though—if anyone finds this, please send it my way!

---

[*] When I emailed Safe Food to enquire about their source, they removed the reference. Meat & Wine Co. never replied.

Opinion vs. Facts

Emotive language often signifies opinions, whereas facts should be stated plainly and backed up by credible sources. Facts can be verified, while an opinion is subject to interpretation and change. Also, look for absolutes: words like 'definitely', 'cause' or 'prove'. A key component of good quality science is that it knows it can never 'prove' anything. Science is rigorous, it follows procedures, and it can find correlations and potential causes, but scientists know that they can never say something is 100% certain, as there's always a margin of error. With statistical analysis, there's always the possibility that the opposite could be true. A true scientist will use words like 'may', 'probably', 'most likely', or 'to the best of our knowledge', but will never use 'this proves that...' or 'this definitely causes...' or any similar statement of certainty. If someone is either using this type of definitive language or calling out another author for not being definitive enough, it's a clear sign that they're not scientifically trained.

This would be a good time to let you know about another catchphrase of the scientific community: 'Correlation does not equal causation.' This means that two things may seem to happen together, but without a controlled test, we cannot say without a doubt that one thing causes the other. They may not even be related! Just because shark attacks happen to increase when ice cream sales go up doesn't mean that eating ice cream makes you tasty to sharks—more likely, there's a third factor influencing both things, like hot sunny days meaning more people in the water and more people desiring an icy refreshment. The two things could be totally random too, such as the weird correlation between Nicolas

Chapter 8: Get Educated

Cage films and swimming pool drownings[4]. The internet is both amazingly wonderful and astonishingly odd...

Results

The way results are displayed visually, such as graphs and charts, can be used for influence, too. Reporting results faithfully in a published study requires that values in charts start at zero and include all data, whereas news articles will often zoom in on a particular part of the chart to make a small difference seem bigger than it really is. As an example, see Figure 13, in which the true chart starting at zero and showing a negligible change (A) can be made to seem much more dramatic than it really is (B), when they've zoomed in. Check carefully though—sometimes they might start at zero but then use a // somewhere along the axis to skip over a significant chunk of values.

Visual influence in graphs

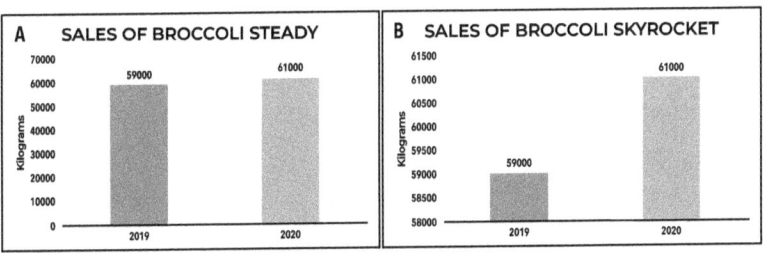

(Fictional data)

Figure 13. Comparison of the Same Data Reported Faithfully or With Visual Influence (Fictional Data)

Another one to look out for is when talking percentages—for example, 'Eating Broccoli Increases Libido By 50%' (this is made up data). An *absolute* percentage means that it would have increased by 50 percentage points, say from 5% to 55%, whereas *relative* percentage would have increased by 50% (half) of the original number, say from 5% to 7.5%. News reports will very rarely define what percentage they're using, but you should know that it's usually *relative,* because it's easy to make small increments sound impressive. (In other words, if something doubles, it might only have gone from 1% to 2%.)

Context
After evaluating the merits of the content, we need to look at it within the big picture. The context in which a piece is published can tell us a lot about potential bias. Does your article come from a reputable scientific journal, or from a tabloid news website? Is it a video from a nutrition conference, or from a foodie channel? Most individual pieces of content will be written from one perspective and have many assumptions about what you, as the reader, already know and believe. The author may also not have the knowledge (or intent) to explore all facets of the problem they're talking about. An article published in an agricultural journal about the biodiversity of pasture-raised cattle is unlikely to focus on the moral considerations of eating animals or the health risks associated with red meat. Just because it's not mentioned doesn't mean it doesn't exist, and omission is often a clever tactic on the part of the author. It's always smart to ask, 'What's *not* being said?'

Also have a think about the history of the time when it was published. Have our general knowledge or societal values changed since then? In my recent university course, we had a unit that explored scientific racism in Indigenous

Australia. Peer-reviewed articles from the 1950s were published in respected medical journals, but they used terminology that would be deemed derogatory now, and modern science has since disproven those old theories. Books and popular culture produced around that time would also be considered out of touch with our modern lens, but it was likely very acceptable back then. On the flip side of out-of-date research, check whether your piece fits with current understanding and is backed up by existing research on the topic. If it's completely leftfield and new, there's probably a lot of questions unanswered, and more research is needed before we can make any claims.

Hierarchy of Evidence

Along with evaluating the content of the piece, it's also key to understand where it sits on the hierarchy of evidence. With science, some types of research are better than others when it comes to the strength of their statements and results[5]. There's no hard and fast rule; if you google this, you'll see pyramids with various descriptions for each of the layers, but the general order goes like this, from best to least:

Meta-Analyses and Systematic Reviews
The best style of evidence is usually meta-analyses or systematic reviews. These research papers critically evaluate and analyse results from a breadth of previous experiments and studies, and they combine a total body of literature on the topic. These types of studies collate and synthesise the research, which avoids relying on the results of only one study that may have

been biased or poorly designed. They're an invaluable part of any professional's ongoing education, because there literally aren't enough hours in the day for each individual to read every single new paper that's published in their field. Industry guidelines and professional recommendations, such as medical treatments, are often created from these types of studies. If you've come across a peer-reviewed meta-analysis, you can be fairly confident that you're seeing an accurate evaluation of the total evidence on this topic.

Randomised Control Trials (RCT)
These are often referred to as the gold standard of research. When they're well-designed with minimal variables, reduced bias, control groups, and double-blind tests, they can test a hypothesis and develop conclusions based around cause and effect. Importantly though, we still can't say they give 'proof' because there's always a margin of statistical error. RCTs are the strongest experimental design, but they can't always be used for ethical reasons, and sometimes an observational/cohort study (next in the list) will provide stronger evidence for outcomes. For example, although there have been thousands of cohort studies on smoking, there's never been an RCT to demonstrate that smoking causes lung cancer, as it would be unethical to force some people to smoke and not others. Diet is also something that's better understood by cohort studies, as RCTs can usually only evaluate one element or ingredient during a short time frame, and that's just not how we eat in real life.

Chapter 8: Get Educated

Observational/Cohort Studies
Following a group of people over time to monitor outcomes, these studies can be much larger and provide thousands of data points, such as the EPIC-Oxford studies. Huge studies evaluating diet and lifestyle outcomes can show strong correlation between variables (such as eating veggies and reduced heart attacks) and can find patterns, but they still can't say that one thing caused the other. Even though they can't find cause, they can sometimes be more powerful than RCTs due to large sample sizes: a 20-year study of 10,000 people across five countries can provide a lot more evidence than a two-week RCT of 46 people in one city.

Case Studies
These are excellent for really diving deep into the lived experience of an individual or small group of people. Case studies are used to explore the details, and they're a starting point for producing ideas and theories to then run further experiments on. Generally, we're not able to extrapolate these results to the general public. Case-controlled studies conducted by professional researchers generally involve hypothesis testing, standardised evaluations, and statistical analysis, and are therefore very different from personal anecdotal stories (which are further down the list).

Animal Studies
While RCTs can be performed on animals, the main reason animal studies are much further down this list is simple: animals are not humans. Although we're similar and share many genetics, our physiology is different to the animals we

test on. Animal behaviours and genetics even differ from species to species, and since we humans are only another species of mammal, we cannot make assumptions about the effect on humans based on what happens in animal trials. This is a strong argument to get rid of animal testing altogether, since it's not even that good quality[6]. Be very careful using or relying on evidence that comes from animal trials, especially with regards to nutrition.

Anecdotes/Opinions
Whether written as an open letter in a well-respected academic journal, or uploaded to a blog, YouTube video or Facebook post, anecdotes and opinions are simply that. While personal stories may be moving and memorable, they're not scientific evidence because variables are not controlled (like in a study), which means that their results cannot be transferable to a wider population.

There's also no way of validating the information. Be careful of the stories that start with, 'I knew a guy who...' or 'My grandmother ate/smoke/drank that, and she lived to 90.' All these stories may be true, but they don't represent the experience for the majority, especially when higher quality science demonstrates otherwise. When a high-quality study finds that eating broccoli does not, in fact, increase libido in 98% of people, there are still 2% of people that may experience a surge, so to speak, so of course we're going to hear stories from the outliers—they're interesting and they capture the imagination.

When it comes to health, anything moving away from the mainstream Western diet is generally going to improve

Chapter 8: Get Educated

quality of life. So while someone may say how eating red meat has been the best thing they've done for their skin, we need to assess where they came from and what they were eating before they changed their diet. Even when written by scientists and experts in their field, opinion pieces can be compelling, but they aim to inspire thinking (and funding) for the future direction of research—they're not science themselves. Stories can be inspirational, but they can't be compared to rigorous science.

As you can see, you don't need to have a science degree or be a research professional to learn a couple of key skills when it comes to investigating your information. You can also use this to evaluate the arguments that others are presenting to you. Rather than firing back your own truth, you can ask them questions to identify the source of *their* information, and this may be enough to unravel their argument and make them begin questioning for themselves. That's a useful skill of influence. Having high-quality evidence to back up facts and provide strong cases will help you to challenge what is generally accepted as truth for the majority of people.

Why Doesn't the Media Tell Us the Truth?

If it's so important to provide credible research, why isn't the truth all over the media? Simple: the media thrives on confusion. They make profit by attracting eyeballs, and eyeballs are attracted to what's new and interesting. We're wired to pay attention to novel things and to ignore what we've already acknowledged. The truth about healthy living doesn't change, so if the media were to consistently share the same story about whole foods and regular exercise, we'd tune out. Instead, it's in their interest to constantly have a new fad or craze to talk about. They love new research and unique case studies: not to learn something new, but to tell us something different. As a consumer, please beware of headlines. They're designed to be emotive, controversial, and sensationalist. Dig deeper—you may need to do your own research to learn how the study is conducted, by whom, if the findings translate to humans, and how it fits with current science. One study doesn't create a breakthrough, no matter what the headline says. It still needs to be replicated and verified. Scientific understanding is built out over decades.

Using Your Newfound Power of Knowledge

Part of educating myself was overcoming my own biases and letting go of the desire to 'see for myself'. Growing up in Australia, I'd only ever seen cows grazing on green fields, and 'happy' animals at the Royal Show. But just because I've never seen a factory farm with 20,000 chickens crammed into a barn full of toxic fumes doesn't mean they don't exist. Just because I haven't seen with my own eyes the destruction of the Amazon doesn't mean it isn't happening. If I relied on only my own experience for everything in life, I wouldn't make it very far.

It's essential to be able to learn from others. If Einstein also had to figure out the law of gravity instead of relying on Isaac Newton's experiments, he wouldn't have had time to develop his Theory of Relativity. We all stand on the shoulders of giants. An early self-help book taught me that we don't have time to make all the mistakes ourselves: we have to learn from others. We have to build on the evidence that came before. We have to know that it's good quality and trustworthy evidence

Chapter 8: Get Educated

that can provide a foundation for what comes next. We don't have time to travel to all these places and see for ourselves with our own eyes (nor do we have the legal clearance to go rooting around farmers' private chicken farms), which is why we need to know about critically evaluating information so that we can know what's truth and what's marketing.

On the other hand, using my own lived experience *is* best, however, when it comes to my own health. Knowing which foods work for my body, what I need to be able to stick to habits, how I support my mental health...all this is personal. While I can get advice from the results of scientific studies and see what *might* work for *most* people, I still need to try it out for myself. Juice cleansing, cold showers, and walks in the morning really work for me; apple cider vinegar, 97% dark chocolate, and whale noises while I'm trying to sleep do *not*, unfortunately (although others may swear by them). You gotta try these things for yourself to know for sure. The benefit of knowing how to find good-quality evidence sources is that I can make informed decisions about where to start, to find what works for me as an individual.

Undertaking research and doing some trial and error is needed to know what works for you, but that doesn't mean that you need to do it alone. One of the best ways to get educated about yourself is to work with professionals like nutritionists and dietitians who have specialised education in the field. Those who specialise in plant-based nutrition and are ideally thriving on a plant-based diet themselves can speak not only from a medical standpoint but also from personal experience. For my first three months of transitioning to the vegan diet, I worked with an amazing dietitian in Brisbane who was a great example of this. While she wasn't completely plant-based herself because eating too many beans didn't agree with her digestion (and I think that many of us can empathise, to be honest), she was able to give me real advice about what specific foods to try, even sending me screenshots of the actual product to buy in Woolies*.

A note of caution: your regular GP isn't necessarily the best source of advice for nutrition. This isn't because they're deceptive or biased, but because of all the 'general' knowledge they've been armed with to treat patients in a broader sense, which means that they're usually not specialised in diet. In fact, nutrition might be only one unit of a four-year degree, and perhaps not even mandatory. Your GP can be a great first point of contact to refer you to other specialists, such as dietitians, and also to mental health professionals, like psychologists. (Going vegan is about more than the food: we may need mindset support, too.) With any professional you engage, check their experience, their education, and their credibility.

~

So, what to do now with all this education you've gathered? Maybe it's just for your own knowledge so that you can make the best decisions that are right for you. Maybe you'll be called to share what you know, whether that's creating a podcast,

---

* AKA 'Woolworths', which is one of our common supermarket chains in Australia. Think of Tesco, Walmart, Aldi, or wherever you shop for groceries. (And no, it doesn't sell koala feed or dingo bait.)

Chapter 8: Get Educated

writing a book, or getting into activism. Or it might be as simple as preparing yourself with responses to the myriad of questions you're bound to be asked by family and friends.

When people hear that I'm vegan, they often seem compelled to mention something that they've heard about, such as, 'Yeah, but heaps of rodents die in crop deaths, so even vegans kill animals', and now that I know how to answer that, I feel confident saying, 'That's true, and can I tell you something interesting about that?'* Ed Winters (AKA Earthling Ed) has a great guide with vegan responses to 30 common (and perhaps exhausting) questions, and his popular Ted Talk claims to bust all vegan myths in 17 minutes. See the resource list at the end of this book.

However, don't feel like you have to learn everything about *all* the topics related to veganism. It's not your job to be the expert, and it can be overwhelming to try and keep up. People come into this vegan world for many different reasons, and once you start exploring, you see how everything is connected—even issues as seemingly far removed as migrant workers, fast fashion, ocean dead zones, and first-world privilege. Vegans and non-vegans alike will have different connotations about what's involved in the vegan lifestyle, and they'll each have different questions based on what's important to *them*. For your own sanity, it's vital to understand that not all arguments are yours. You don't have to attend every heated discussion you're

---

* For your reference, I answer this from two angles: 1) There's a huge difference between intentional slaughter and accidental harvest deaths, like bugs on a windshield, and 2) Animals need to eat way more crops than humans do, so by eliminating animal feed, we're actually saving many lives of rodents because we'll be farming less crops.

invited to. Just because you care deeply about eliminating animal suffering doesn't mean that you also know everything about climate change. Just because you may be fighting for the survival of our planet doesn't mean that you also know everything about animal abuse and human rights issues. Just because you embrace this way of life doesn't mean that you're the authority on it (not yet, anyway).

My friend and vegan inspiration, Belinda, has a story about a time when she was abused by a complete stranger for not being 'vegan enough'. During an off-roading trip, she was fuelling up her 4WD, and when she came out of the kiosk, a lady was standing behind her car reading her bumper stickers about animal rights and being vegan. The lady started yelling at her that she shouldn't be driving a gas-guzzling 4WD, because of the environmental damage, if she claims to be vegan. Belinda, as a member of the Animal Justice Party, knows all about animal rights, is an outspoken activist, and is planning on building her own rescue farm. Yet she openly admits that she doesn't spend as much time learning about the environmental impact or the healthy food options. She's vegan for the animals and that's her passion. But so many of us want to crucify others for not completely walking the talk. Give me a break! Again, don't accept every debating invitation that you receive.

Each of us has our own passions, and we only have so much energy to fight for our own cause. If all of us focused on the issues we were respectively passionate about, we'd solve everything, because someone else will always care about the topics that you don't. Not that you don't care at all, just not enough to give up your weekends for it. If everyone in the whole world was vegan for the animals and only cared about eliminating their suffering, who would be focused on sweatshops, ocean clean-up, food waste, child labour, reducing crime, prisoner rehabilitation, sexism, racism, mental health support, suicide prevention, and all the other issues in this world that need addressing? I might be biased when I say that vegans are pretty powerful, but even *I'll* admit that we can't solve everything. That's why the militant vegans are so great—they're fighting for animal justice, and we need them to keep going. The rest of the world might not be passionate enough to attend rallies and rescue animals, but they don't need to do that to still make a difference. Whatever your mission is, just eat plants while you do it. Reducing demand for meat, dairy, and eggs will go a long way to making a dent in the most serious issue of our species: the survival of our home planet*.

Now, armed with evidence and the skills to evaluate new information, you can support yourself as you transition to a plant-based way of life.

---

* I realise that I said 'home planet' as if there's another one we can move to. Reminder: there's not.

CHAPTER 9: Allow the Transition

When I was little, I had dreams of playing the piano. My parents even rented one so that I could learn at home. I did some lessons and practised a couple of songs, but when I wasn't good at it right away, I quit. I've never gone back to the piano (although I can still play that right-hand part of 'Heart & Soul') and sometimes I wonder: If I'd stuck with it, would I be performing in shows and selling out concert halls by now? Did I miss the boat for my virtuoso destiny?

I'm sure I'm not the only one who's given up on something because it got too hard. Our childhood closets are crammed with guitars, ballet shoes, and astronaut costumes. Deciding to be vegan can be a similar situation. At first, it's exciting and we throw ourselves into it, but when we get invited to a camping trip or our niece's birthday party or have to deal with all the questions and challenges (from literally everyone from Mum to the lady at the bookstore), things can start to

Chapter 9: Allow the Transition

unravel, especially if we're not prepared.

I know now that you can't expect to master the piano overnight. Even if you do your research and know which fingers to use for which keys, you still need to learn the language of reading music, practice so that you build up the muscle memory, and get used to the nerves that come with performing in front of other people. It's similar when you go vegan: you need time to research alternative food options, practice making meals that taste good, and build up your confidence dealing with people out there in the world. Even if you were able to magically read all the books and watch all the documentaries in one night, you still need to practice the habits that will sustain you over time.

Being vegan is a lifestyle, not a quick diet to drop five kilos and save three animals. Most of us who choose this way of living want to be able to commit to it for a lifetime. It's linked to our morals, and we want to pass on this philosophy to future generations, too. But it's also an absolutely huge undertaking—not only turning our whole life around but doing so while living in a carnist society that wants us to maintain the status quo. We need to have strong habits to keep us on track.

When it comes to habits, most of us do what we do just because we do it. (Read that sentence again—it actually does make sense, and it's really something to ponder). Habits are who we are. For someone who follows the mainstream diet, it could be the habit of snacking on a chunk of cheddar cheese, or automatically choosing bacon and eggs for breakfast, or the easy mental math of calculating protein intake based on the weight of meat.

Habits come from a neurological loop based on triggers and rewards. We see, hear, or feel something as a cue, we get a craving, and we take action until the craving is satisfied. For me, I walk past the cinema, I smell popcorn, and I want popcorn. If I don't go in straight away and buy a tub to take home (yes, I do that), then I'll probably end up saying to Phil, 'Hey, let's go to the movies later.' Satisfying the craving releases neurochemicals like dopamine that link the good feeling to the original cue, and so the cycle continues. The 'craving' that we satisfy could be simply taking the easy option or the default route—the outcome of our lazy brains. Habits can definitely be broken, and new ones can be formed, but this doesn't happen overnight.

Another reason we find it so hard to change habits is because they're linked to our identity. So, as James Clear explains in his book *Atomic Habits*[1], the trick is to redefine how we see ourselves. *Atomic Habits* teaches us that a 1% change makes a huge difference over time, which is why it's okay to focus on getting better every day rather than expecting an overnight miracle. This is the reason why I'm proud of myself for only getting the medium popcorn, not the large one (unless, of course, it's one of those long, three-hour movies, then there's no question).

There are both good and bad things about changing habits around a vegan diet: it's hard because the temptations around our old food are constantly in our face all day every day (especially when living with people who are still enjoying our favourite comfort foods), but this also means that we have so many opportunities to choose something different.

Because we're humans and not robots, it takes time to

Chapter 9: Allow the Transition

change habits, and they need to be incorporated into our life. It's totally fine to start small, with one change at a time. Later in this chapter, we'll identify some simple swaps you could make that can replace existing habits. Or you could explore structured activities like Meat Free Mondays or Veganuary. Veganuary has been running for ten years now, and research shows that 30% of participants continue the vegan diet after January and 82% maintain a reduction in demand for animal products, because they've built some habits and found some easy meals to fit into their life[2]. You also don't need to wait until January to begin—companies like VeganEasy have a free, 30-day vegan challenge you can start any time.

If you can't, or don't want to, be a full-time vegan, other options are being 'flexitarian' or 'vegan before 6pm' or 'vegan except for Sundays'. Whichever way you do it, it's got to be sustainable and practical for you. Some very strict vegans take the pledge in which they wear a fork bracelet and refuse to sit at any table where animal products are served. I admire their commitment, but it's not something that's feasible for me, especially being in a mixed-veg relationship. Also, I don't know how I feel about wearing a kitchen utensil on my wrist.

While data shows that the best diet for the climate of our planet is 100% plant-based—and it goes without saying by now that it's also best for the animals—you don't need to be 'all or nothing' for the health benefits (this was covered earlier, but it bears reinforcing). There's no science (to date) saying that we need to eat 100% plants: remember, the benefits are gained from 85% onwards, which matches up with the EAT-Lancet recommendation of 88% plant-based for a global diet to sustain our planet. Even our Blue Zones with the highest concentration of healthy 100-year-olds continue to eat small amounts of meat or dairy. That final 12-15% gives you the flexibility to shift and transition without feeling like giving up because it's all too hard[3,4].

For me, eating at home makes it easy to be vegan, but eating out can often be a challenge. I'll usually plan ahead and check out the menus, but sometimes we end up somewhere and they've only got vegetarian options. I'll see if they can amend it, but if not, I'll be vegetarian for that meal. And I won't sweat it.

Remember that the key is consistency, not perfection. Being flexible is smart: it's sustainable over the long term, better for your mental health, and more inspiring to those around you, because they'll see how they can come along on the journey, too. Allowing yourself to transition with small changes and adaptations over time is going to be more sustainable and more beneficial for the world in the long run. This is something that needs to last a lifetime, so wherever you are in your transition or exploration of this vegan lifestyle, below are some ideas of simple habit swaps you can make.

Mince meat
Basically any recipe that calls for mince will be suitable for lentils instead. Lentils are full of fibre, protein, iron, and heaps of other good stuff, and they have a similar texture and 'meatiness', which makes the dish feel the same. I use lentils in casseroles, savoury mince, tacos, and bolognaise, to name just a smattering of options. The key is seasonings. It's not the taste of the dead animal flesh that we like, it's the spices and condiments in the dish. So if you get the seasoning right—and

Chapter 9: Allow the Transition

it's easy to do with thousands of recipes online—then you've got an environmentally friendly, cruelty-free, and healthy meal option.

Steak

Okay, this won't *taste* like steak, but a good option to replace the fillet of steak or chicken at dinner time is a veggie patty. It serves the same purpose on a plate: you cut a bit off, add some mashed potato and veggies to your fork, dunk it in the gravy, and let your tastebuds go wild. Since my husband hasn't joined me on my vegan journey (yet!), I often make a meal for us, but give him steak while I have a veggie patty. Different taste, but it means we eat together with the same side dishes. Works for roast dinners, BBQs...anything where the meat is served on its own next to the sides—and there are heaps of patty options in both the fridge and freezer section of the supermarket.

What About Seitan for Steak?

Yes, seitan does look a lot more like steak, especially with the right chargrill coating. The first time I ate it as a meal (actually, I think it's the only time), I managed to get through half a steak, with a generous forkful of fries and salad in each bite. For a meat eater, it really does look like steak, so the brain starts to prepare for what it expects (have you ever heard that we 'eat with our eyes'?), but the doughy, chewy texture just really threw me off. Phil even tried some—and then promptly spat it out. Yes, in the restaurant. But if you can get past the texture, it's a good quality source of protein, and also minimally processed. It just didn't make it into my top recommendations for the texture reason.

Chicken breast

Instead of chicken in my salad or wraps, I've been using tofu. Firm tofu that's pre-marinated can be bought from the shops, so it's a couple of minutes to fry up (no pressing necessary) and then I slice or dice it for whatever suits the meal. And it's delicious cold too, so you can batch cook. Okay, it doesn't taste exactly like chicken, but the texture is pretty close, and with the right seasonings, you won't even miss the bird.

Milk

Any alternative milk is better for the environment than dairy[5]. Per litre of milk for consumption, dairy requires 628 litres of water compared to the next-highest plant milk, almond, which uses 371 litres. Oat milk is my favourite since it tastes creamy, and it generates some of the lowest amount of water use (48 litres) and emissions. My recommendation is to choose one that's fortified with calcium, and you can substitute it anywhere you'd use dairy milk.

Butter

There are plenty of dairy-free butters and spreads, right next to the regular stuff in the supermarket. I choose Nuttlex (Nuttlex Buttery, to be exact) and it works great for me. It has a slightly different taste, as does anything when you change brands, but you get used to it really quick. It's a delicious substitute for any time you'd use butter, such as frying, mashed potato, and microwave popcorn.

Egg in cocktails and baking

Check out aquafaba: the water from a can of chickpeas. I know, I know—it sounds gross. It's normally the juice that

Chapter 9: Allow the Transition

gets drained and rinsed away, but trust me on this. I'm yet to try aquafaba in baking (I'm not much of a baker, to my husband's sorrow), but there are thousands of recipes online that use aquafaba for meringues, mousse, pancakes, and more. And I know for sure that they work a treat with homemade cocktails—one tablespoon is enough for two Amaretto Sours in your shaker. Unfortunately, for health and safety reasons, you can't bring your own aquafaba into the bar for them to use in your cocktail, but you *can* ask for it, and many bars will have some. Even the act of asking is demonstrating that there's a demand for it.

Parmesan cheese
Nutritional yeast, also known as 'nooch', is something that took me ages to adopt because it sounded weird, and kind of like an infection (you know what I mean, ladies). But it's a powerhouse of nutrients—protein, fibre, and that ever-elusive vitamin B12—and it *does* taste just like parmesan cheese. I haven't used it yet in baking (see above, complete with hubby's tears), but I liberally sprinkle it over my pasta dishes, and it really hits the spot.

Mayo
There's a vegan version of most sauces and condiments these days from common brands like Heinz, Hellman's, and Praise, so you don't have to go far to find one. But to give a bit of flavour and sauciness to my wraps or salads, I've mostly been using hummus, which also comes in a variety of vegan-friendly flavours. It also has more protein in it, and it isn't as processed as mayo.

The Imperfect Vegan

Burgers
Plenty of restaurants offer veggie burgers, from fancy pubs to fast-food places. If you want to be healthy, you can go for the patty made of actual smooshed-up veggies, or you can treat yourself with Impossible or Beyond patties. These delicious options taste literally like beef mince, so you really don't know you're missing anything. They're still 100% plant-based and have a similar protein/iron nutrient profile to beef, and with the extra benefit of fibre. Even though they're *way* better for the environment than beef, they *are* considered highly processed: they contain high amounts of sodium and are best regarded as a splurge. Check out Grill'd, Carl's Jr., or Burger King, or buy your own burger patties from the supermarket.

Chips/Crisps
You don't need to trek to the specialty store for vegan chips, and they don't need to be weird beet or plantain chips either. (Yes, I said weird. Give me a potato any day.) Plenty of brands have accidentally vegan options, like Doritos original salt, Smith's plain salt, Red Rock salt and vinegar, Pringles BBQ, lots of Lay's flavours, and Ritz crackers. PETA has some great lists for accidentally vegan snack foods on their website. Always check the label in case they change their ingredients.

Ice cream
These days, there are plant-based versions of your favourite brands, including Magnum, Drumstick, Ben & Jerry's, and Connoisseur—often right there in the frozen isle of the supermarket. And no, they're not all made of tofu and coconut: my ice cream snob of a non-vegan husband will happily eat

Chapter 9: Allow the Transition

my salted caramel dairy-free Magnums (whether *I'm* happy about this is a different story).

Chocolate

Okay, so your favourite Cadbury bars will probably have to go, but there are heaps of other delicious options. Whittakers has a couple of naturally vegan options—their Ghana Peppermint and the Rum & Raisin blocks are already vegan. Lindt has brought out a couple of vegan blocks, too. My favourite eco-organic brand of vegan chocolate is Pico: they have a huge variety of flavours, but my go-to is their salted caramel. The Woolies Macro section has a lot of sweet treats, so you'll never be caught short for a chocolate craving.

All these simple swaps are habits that you'll build up over time. Like a muscle, the more you use it, the stronger it gets. The key with a nutritious vegan diet is planning. Don't leave your food shopping until the last minute, try not to order food when you're already starving, and pack snacks if you know you'll be out all day.

If you're not able or ready to make all these food changes yet but you want to continue supporting the movement, below are some other ways you can help:

Skincare

This can be a tricky one to recommend because everyone's skin is so different. But rest assured that there's plenty of vegan skincare brands available, and sometimes the cheap and simple ones are the best, especially for sensitive skin. The less ingredients the better. I recently stopped using expensive Clarins and switched to Simple, the UK brand, which is available in the supermarket and from pharmacy chains like Priceline. Before throwing out your whole collection and buying a brand new one, see if the shop has samples that you can take home to try, and start with one product at a time. (PS—don't listen to the sales reps who tell you that your whole product kit has to come from the same range. They just want their commission.)

Entertainment

Instead of taking the kids to the zoo or SeaWorld, take them to a farm rescue or sanctuary. Farm Animal Rescue is only 45 minutes from Brisbane city, where you can interact with rescued animals living out their natural life, and also enjoy a cruelty-free BBQ. If the ocean is your thing, avoid aquariums and opt for a glass-bottom boat or go diving (just remember the reef-friendly sunscreen). Instead of a circus with animals, make sure it's a people show. When travelling, avoid the caged and drugged tiger sanctuaries and elephant rides, and instead visit rehabilitation reserves or plant trees with the local community.

Food waste

About a third of food produced for humans ends up in waste. If food waste was a country, its land use would make it the second largest one in the world behind Russia; it would equate to the third largest carbon emitter behind the US and China; and it would account for more freshwater use than any other single country[6]. Landfill food is a banquet for the microbes and bacteria that produce methane, which is a far more destructive GHG than carbon. You can help by planning your meals and buying only what you need. Do smaller shops more frequently and use what you've got before it goes off. Get creative in the kitchen and try mixing leftovers together. Smell food before just chucking it out—best before dates are only a guide, and even 'expiry' dates have some leeway. There are plenty of resources online, like stilltasty.com, which can help you determine if it's still good. Of course, use your judgement and always protect your health. No one is asking you to eat rotten food, but a *lot* of the food we throw away is still good, and you'd be better off nourishing your gut than contributing to methane production in a landfill. And think of the money you'll save, too.

Other ways you can reduce food waste include composting at home or finding a local garden that'll gladly take your scraps. Unfortunately, a lot of food waste comes from supermarkets that only want the beautiful fruits and vegs, and the 'ugly' ones end up in the bin. It's crazy, but they're only responding to consumer demand. However, supermarkets often have a section for weirdly shaped items now, such as 'The Odd Bunch' at Woolworths or the 'I'm Perfect' range at Coles. You can also shop at farmers' markets, which generally have all produce available, no matter what shape, size, or colour it is!

Support advocacy or charities
It's not hypocritical to give money to charities that are doing the work you're not able to do—just like it's not hypocritical to eat fully vegan but not go to protests.

Buy ethical meats
This is easier said than done because you need to be wary of the greenwashing, and also of the labels that don't mean what you think they mean. But if you have the time and the

means, get out into the country and find farms that are raising animals in a way that you're comfortable with, and only buy your products from them. A good place to start your research is in local organics or wholefood stores, as they often have meats from high-quality, small-farm suppliers. There's a group of farmers who subscribe to the philosophy of 'one bad day,' meaning that their animals live cruelty-free and humane lives up until, well, the last day of their lives, and that might be something you're comfortable with. But again, do your own research without relying on the fancy labels and websites.

While being vegan comes down to more than just the food, it's usually the reason most people give up, because food is so entwined in every part of our lives. For those who came into veganism for the animals, it might be easy for you to avoid consuming animal products because you can immediately associate it with torture and pain. With this mindset, deciding not to eat meat is the same as deciding not to eat humans, or your dog. It just *is*. Whereas someone who's vegan for environmental reasons might still love the smell of roast lamb and find it a constant struggle to remember the environmental damage, since it can't always be seen right in front of us. Even for those who came to veganism for health reasons will still experience cravings for a convenient chunk of cheddar cheese (the daddy of all cravings for many of us).

These struggles and temptations don't make us hypocrites—they make us human. We all have different ways of dealing. Some people work best with a complete shift, such as throwing out any foods, clothing, cleaning products, and skincare that contain animal products so that they can start

Chapter 9: Allow the Transition

fresh. Others are happy to continue using up the existing ingredients to prevent food waste and will continue using their cosmetics and wearing their clothing until they need replacement, and then choosing the vegan option.

Please don't feel like you have to do it all at once, and never let anyone put pressure on you for how long your transition takes or which parts you're still working on. Everyone is on their own journey, and every step you take towards a more plant-based lifestyle is making a difference in the world.

Whatever path you take, continue to have compassion for yourself. It's okay to take it slow, as long as you keep doing the best you can. When you make mistakes, forgive yourself. When you choose your meals, do so with intention. When you're unable to cut out a certain animal product for whatever reason, continue to educate yourself and look after your health. You're doing a *really* good thing, and it's a big deal. Sometimes it's harder than expected, but the more we all do it, the easier it will be for everyone. And always remember, you're not alone in this. The next chapter will explore how to connect with support to help you along the journey.

CHAPTER 10: Connect with Support

While being vegan is a personal choice and something only you can do for yourself, that doesn't mean you have to do it alone. There's *so* much support out there to help you on your way. Like many people I've spoken with, if we don't have support and someone to talk to, we run the risk of reverting to the mainstream diet because it's just easier, not only socially but mentally as well. And if we do that, we'll always be living with the uncomfortable cognitive dissonance that our actions aren't lining up with our beliefs. The most important step is connecting with our own WHY and getting clear on our reasons for doing this. We also need to find a community to connect with, and build a support network that can include professionals like dietitians and therapists. Throughout all of it, it's important to ignore the haters and look for ways to manage our mixed-veg relationships.

Chapter 10: Connect with Support

No matter where you are, you'll usually find many like-minded people to connect with: if it's not local city groups with in-person meet-ups, there'll be worldwide movements with online chat groups. On Facebook alone, there's recipe-sharing groups, activism communities, and influencers to follow; and in the real world, you can look for groups at university, at work, or in your local community centre.

As with all social connectivity, there are going to be people who get along and others who don't. There'll be big personalities, judgements about moral superiority, unexamined privilege, and also 'in-groups' and 'out-groups'—that's just human nature, and we can't get away from that part of our psychology. Not everyone is going to feel exactly how you feel about the same topic. You might be really keen to eat everything that replicates meat (like Chick'n nuggets), and others might be avoiding those kinds of products because they're processed. Some people might believe that you need to take a stand with everyone you meet and spread the virtues of the movement, and others might just want to eat their veggies in peace without causing a stir. You'll have an opinion about what others are doing, and they'll have an opinion about you. That's the nature of social interaction.

Never feel like you have to stick with a group or join in on things that you're not comfortable with. You don't *have* to go to protests and chain yourself to the gates at chicken farms. You don't *have* to get into an argument with every meat eater you come across. You don't *have* to post pics of your plant-based meals on social media.

There's a lot of judgement in groups, and that's just social nature. We'll get that in any group we join, not just a vegan

The Imperfect Vegan

community. Because being vegan is linked to morals—it's the same as religion in that way—emotions run high and there are passionate zealots who'll try to convert everyone else to their way of thinking. But just like there's no one way to worship whomever or whatever you choose (if at all), there's no one way to be vegan. Who wants boring uniformity anyway?

I know that the militant vegans are fighting for a good cause, and that their morals towards animals are beautiful and fierce. They set the bar for what's possible in this cause. Just like every movement has its hardcore extreme militants, we need them, but we don't need to *be* them, and nor do we need to feel pressured by them. They're leading the way, and we need them to be unwavering in their commitment (and if you're one of these, thank you!). I love that they're so passionate about the animals, but it's unrealistic to think that everyone in the world has the exact same fierce passion for one issue. We all need to have our own enthusiasm because there's lots in the world that needs fixing. For the rest of us who join the vegan movement, we can contribute to the cause by doing the best we can. Never let the purists make you feel bad for not doing enough. They can inspire you to do more of what more you *can* do if it's possible for you, but not a prescription for what you *have* to do. As we've been learning throughout this book, perfection is *not* the goal—sustaining change over the long term and inspiring as many people as possible to reduce their demand on the animal industry is what's going to make the difference.

Even though I've experienced the toxicity of purist vegans in Facebook groups, I've mostly experienced way more support and connection. In my favourite group, people

Chapter 10: Connect with Support

share recommendations for local restaurants, ask for where to get certain vegan foods, discuss what's available in the supermarkets, share news stories, recipes, and promote meet-up groups and local vegan markets. More often than not, the comments are supportive, and we love to shout out local vegan businesses—what a great way to learn about and support small companies that are contributing to our new way of living. For me, this has been a place where I can feel validated, get inspired and ask questions, especially since most of my real-world relationships are 'mixed veg'.

~

It's probably obvious what I mean by a mixed-veg relationship, but to clarify, I apply the term to any relationship, such as a romantic partnership, in which one person is vegan and the other isn't, or to two people who are different types of veg, like vegan and vegetarian. It also applies to families—I'm the only vegan in my immediate family, although one of my aunts has been vegetarian since she was a teenager.

Relationships can also apply to any situation, like getting lunch with your colleagues at work or the end-of-year event with your football group. Let's face it—pretty much everything in life is both social and food-oriented. In social, food-based events like Christmas and Thanksgiving, there's a lot more going on than the food being served. There's meaning behind the occasion. There's tradition, stories, and connection. It's all tied up together, and not always easy to separate.

In these situations, you've got to do what's right for you. If you're vegan all year round and you choose to eat the turkey once a year to keep the peace with your family who you never see otherwise, you may decide it's no big deal. Or you could choose to cater for yourself and bring your own food and vegan wine. You could offer to cook a couple of vegan dishes or offer to host at your place and do all the cooking. (If so, make sure to pick your best-tasting, tried-and-tested meals. Christmas dinner is not the time to experiment with a new dish, no matter how many five-star ratings it has.) If you refuse to sit at the table where animals are consumed, you could arrive later and join them after the meal. One of our activists in Australia, Joey Carbstrong, put out a great video last year sharing three types of vegans and ways that each of them might deal with Christmas dinner[1]. Remember, the best action is whatever works for *you*.

In relationships with others, there's never a clear-cut solution or answer. Even social psychologists spend decades in research to understand human behaviour and what drives us, and they can still only come up with theories and best estimates. *You* are the one who knows your relationships, and *you* are the one who has to live the situation. By all means, get ideas and advice from people you trust and respect, but never feel like you *have* to do anything a certain way. Just because one loud vegan in your Facebook group has an opinion doesn't mean that everyone needs to follow suit. Each situation can be different, and the way you respond this time might be different to next time (remember how humans are walking contradictions?). It's okay to change your mind. You're not a robot. You're not a hypocrite for doing it differently, and you don't need to be perfect at this.

Sometimes when Phil goes to the bottle shop, I follow

Chapter 10: Connect with Support

him around with my Barnivore app at the ready and tell him whether the wine he picked up is vegan or not, and other times I leave him in peace. Sometimes I suggest to bar owners that they should identify their vegan wines on the menu, and other times I just enjoy the fact they even had a wine for me to enjoy. We don't have to try and convert everyone we come into contact with.

When I do want to talk about it, I've learnt to leave emotions and judgement to the side. Although I must admit I'm not perfect at this either. Show me someone who *is*, right? My aim is always to listen to the other person first—I try to remember one of Steven Covey's *Seven Habits*[2], 'Seek First to Understand', and so I'll ask questions, explore their thinking, and put myself in their shoes. I've also learnt to choose my timing. Non-vegans feel most defensive about their beliefs when they're eating or have just eaten animal products[3]. In that moment, our brains are in high activity to justify and rationalise our actions.

You may also become the subject of interrogation by non-vegans, without you even saying anything. Just your act of choosing a vegan meal can trigger their own defences, and they'll want to assuage their cognitive dissonance. Some people are genuinely curious, like Shea who saw that I ordered a vegan burrito after our run club, and told me how much she admired what I was doing because she wasn't able to commit fully herself (Shea has the low-iron issue I mentioned in Chapter 4). Others might not be so pleasant, so remember: you never have to stay in a situation you're uncomfortable with. If emotions run high, remove yourself. It also helps to have some common responses ready (like we covered in Chapter

8) or be prepared with topics for changing the subject.

Many vegans I've spoken with say that dealing with relationships is the hardest part, especially with close family. Ed Winters in *Vegan Propaganda* shares that he talks about veganism more with dairy farmers than with his own family, and it's disappointing that the family he loves and most wants to be vegan are defending meat eating to his face.

When you care about someone the most, it's then that you'll more likely forget to be calm and unemotional. The reason I suggest planning ahead so that you don't accidentally say something mean is because I've got an example of when I got this really, really wrong.

I was having a casual lunch with the family: Mum, Dad, my sister, and her two kids. It was a warm sunny day, and we'd stopped at a local café to sit at their outdoor tables. Our family loves to share food, so we were talking about our choices and trying each other's dishes. I don't remember whether it was health or environmental concerns that prompted this, but Mum said, 'That's why I'm eating salmon, because fish isn't so bad, I don't think.' Knowing what I do about the fishing industries, I had a different opinion. Out of my desire to be helpful, what I *meant* to say was, 'I can see why you believe that, and I thought so too at first. If you're curious, I can share with you some of the things I've learned about fish? But only if you ask me, because I won't bombard you about it if you don't want to know.' Nice, right?

What actually came out of my mouth was, 'I can educate you if you like, or you can continue living in ignorance?'

Yes. Those were the actual words out of my mouth. I'm still cringing now.

Chapter 10: Connect with Support

What a wanky, rude, insensitive thing to say. Especially now that I know how times of eating are when people are most defensive. I still feel terrible about it. Of *course* she thinks that fish aren't so bad—recall all that marketing we uncovered in Part 1? Unless you're someone with a vested interest in the topic and have access to information, why would you spend time investigating the opposite of what you already believe?

I stewed on it for a few days, and when I apologised to Mum later, she didn't even seem to remember it. She may have been sparing my feelings (our family is pretty good at avoiding emotional confrontation), but it goes to show that if close relationships are important to you, it's worth investing time in preparing what to say when the topic comes up.

There's no one perfect solution to any of these situations. As relationships with others (and even your own beliefs) develop and mould over time, it's a constant process of decision making and learning. You may decide that for the sake of your mental health, you need to leave relationships that don't align with your beliefs or aren't at least supportive of yours. Many people I've spoken with have chosen to let go of friends and even family for these reasons. But never allow yourself to be pressured to stay or to go—you must do what works for you.

With my husband Phil, we're growing together. I have a clear memory from the start of our relationship when we met two of his friends who were a couple: she was vegan and he wasn't. They seemed happy and close, but I remember saying to Phil that I'm so glad that neither of us is vegan, because I felt it would be too hard and we wouldn't feel like a couple. Shoot forward to five years later and there I go, making the decision to be vegan without him. When I decided to be vegan, I made the choice purely because it felt right inside my bones, like it was the right thing to do. However, I also realised how hard it is to know something so clearly and feel it so deeply, and not understand how someone you love and care about doesn't feel the same way. It was a mental shift I had to get my head around.

I'll be honest: At first, I did question whether I could stay in a relationship with someone whose morals didn't line up with mine. We were already different in many aspects of life: I'm a morning person, he's a night owl; he's very pragmatic, I'm quite a woo-woo; I do CrossFit, he does regular gym. I felt like we'd grow further apart.

Luckily, we have strong communication in our relationship and it helped to talk things through, but the thing that really made the difference was my own mindset. I had to remind myself that everyone is different and that no one is perfect. He's his own person, and he has to make the decisions that are right for him. He has his own priorities, beliefs, and knowledge, and even if they're different to mine, that doesn't mean they're wrong for him. At this time in his life, it's not a priority to research what happens to animals, nor to dig into the damage being done to the environment. Health is a priority and time is a pressure, and he's got his routines with food and knows what works for his own goals. There's those habits in action. Although he may still be able to achieve those goals on plant-based foods, it's not convenient for him right now to try it out. And I have to be okay with that, because I was the same for the first 35 years of my life. I had many vegan friends who tried to tell me about *Cowspiracy* and other things that

Chapter 10: Connect with Support

were happening, but I didn't want to know because I didn't want to have to change my life around. I now thank those friends for not being pushy about it—and it's probably why we're still friends now.

What my husband *does* do is support me—but I know he wouldn't support me as much if I didn't first support his decisions. It's hard to do, mentally, but it's the best mindset shift I've been able to make. My belief is that I'll be an inspiration to him, cooking up delicious meals, making it seem easy, and glowing with health and energy, and then one day he may decide to explore more. He's already reduced his meat intake, he's quite happy to eat my spicy bean chili and fresh buddha bowls (which I'm pleased about too, as long as he doesn't eat the last serving), and he'll take me to plant-exclusive restaurants every now and then, but I love him for who he is, and I won't dictate what he chooses to put on his own plate. And he exercises the same courtesy for me.

When it comes to trying to change people, anyone who's raised a teenager (or been one) will know that the more you force, the more they do the opposite, and that's not something people grow out of. You just have to let go of control and trust that good people will work it out for themselves. Why would I spend my energy trying to convert one person when I can write a book to inspire (hopefully) millions? I'll save my energy for loving my husband where he's at.

This mindset shift is important, because the most powerful system of support is within yourself. It's *essential* to know how to support yourself. No matter the friends and family you're surrounded by now, *you* are the only person you'll be with for the rest of your life. *You* are the only person you need to make happy. When you're living aligned with your values and being true to your heart, everything just flows easier. Yes, there will be bumps in the road and challenges to overcome, but when you're coming from a place of internal belief, and you're connected with your own WHY, those challenges are worthwhile, and you'll have the perseverance you need to get through them.

We're fighting for something really big. Similar to the feminist movement, anti-racism, and ending poverty, these are things that cannot be achieved in one person's lifetime.

Right now, we have many very passionate people fighting for this cause, but it's also starting to become something that's 'cool'—and that's a good thing. Although some purist vegans call it 'virtue signalling' and reject the use of the word 'vegan' outside of the original context of avoiding animal exploitation, I believe that it's going to help the movement. The more people who choose plant-based products, the easier it will be for everyone. It signals to companies that we want vegan brands, and so they'll become more accessible in shops and restaurants. Cosmetics will be plant-based by default. Imagine how great it will be once companies need to clearly label that their products 'contain animal derivatives'—shopping as a vegan will be so much quicker without needing to refer to Google every five seconds.

The problem is that when things are popular, many people will join the movement without a clear sense of why they're in it, besides wanting to be part of the crowd. And this is where it'll get hard. If we don't have a clear WHY—for *anything* that we do, be it starting a business, going to university, or

Chapter 10: Connect with Support

choosing a diet—it's so much harder to stick with it.

As we've explored, people do come into veganism from many different angles, and that's okay. Once we're in, we hear about all the other stuff going on and we feel a sense of obligation to be outraged by all of it. But, like we've learned, not everyone has the same passions. What keeps me up at night, ruminating and worrying about, is the destruction of the environment. What happens if we become climate migrants? What if we lose our house to rising sea levels? What if all the shipping ports are flooded and we can no longer transport food around the world? What if we have to go back to eating off the land? I won't be able to have a balanced diet then, I won't be able to get my creatine, and I certainly won't be able to go to CrossFit. I like my life, it's comfortable. I don't want to have to move, live off the land, or struggle to find water. And then I remember that I'm so frickin' lucky to live in Australia, and that other people around the world are *already* experiencing this. It's not fair that I get to be so comfortable when others don't. The least I can do is watch what I eat so that I don't make it worse. And the second least I can do is write this book and talk about the topic, which will maybe plant a seed that inspires other people to help the cause, too.

That's *my* WHY—it doesn't have to be yours, though. You may feel similar, or you may not. But whatever reason you came into veganism, that's the WHY you need to connect with. If it's important to you, you'll make the switch easier. You'll commit and keep working. All different reasons are valid, so deep dive to understand why *you're* making this choice. What will it give you? What will it do for your life, for the people around you, and for your people in the future? When you get clear on your reasons, you can have a statement ready and prepared when someone asks you, which will make you feel even *more* confident. A clear statement can help others make the connection, too.

Without a strong WHY, it's easy to get trapped again in carnism and to feel like the small actions you take every day aren't important, especially in mainstream society. One of the ways I keep my WHY strong is to keep it 'topped up'. Occasionally, I'll re-watch documentaries like *Forks Over Knives*, *Dominion*, or *Eating Our Way to Extinction* to keep the knowledge fresh. I'll always watch the new ones, and I love to follow activists online to hear the latest research and see what people are talking about now. I've shared some of my favourite resources in the back of this book.

Keep in mind, though, that many of these can be distressing, and I'm not recommending that you stay in a constant state of emotional turmoil. Overexposure to traumatic and graphic material can trigger stress and even lead to PTSD[5]. Instead, you could do simple things like write your WHY on a Post-it and stick it around the house, make a vision board that represents your beliefs, or create a wallpaper for your phone.

Whichever way you connect with yourself and with the people around you is totally up to you. At times it may serve you to completely withdraw from social vegan spaces, and other times they may be your source of strength. Even though there are people in your life who are not on the same journey as you, you can love them anyway for where they're at (and remember that you were once there, too). You may want to try and convince your loved ones to join you. I know I did—and still do—but I learnt that arguing and nit-picking and bombarding them with facts (especially when they're

Chapter 10: Connect with Support

eating—sorry, Mum) isn't the approach that works.

You can't force people to change, but you might be able to inspire them.

CHAPTER 11: Be the Lighthouse

Remember that famous line from the deli scene in *When Harry Met Sally*? Meg Ryan was very exuberantly expressing her pleasure ('Oh, *yes*. Oh, YES!'), turning heads and inspiring another customer to request, 'I'll have what *she's* having.' This line struck such a chord with audiences that it inspired many spin-off ads, such as for Herbal Essences shampoo and Kellogg's cereal. That's what I'm talking about when I advise you to be the lighthouse: exhibit such joy and pleasure in whatever you're doing that other people can't help but take notice and be inspired.

On a slightly grander scale than shampoo, Mahatma Gandhi was a lighthouse: 'Be the change you wish to see' was the motto he gave the world. He travelled throughout India on foot, serving the poor, and leading a movement for Indian independence. Living by example inspired others to join his

Chapter 11: Be the Lighthouse

campaign of non-violence, simplicity, and self-rule.

You don't need to be Gandhi to inspire change, though—you just need to love what you're doing. That's another reason to not put pressure on yourself to be perfect: if it's constantly hard work and stressful, why would anyone aspire to join you? No one wants to hop onto a bandwagon that looks to be a hard slog.

It's part of human nature that feelings are contagious. Have you ever laughed just because someone else had the giggles? Have you ever come home to your partner in a bad mood and instantly felt the low vibes? We actually have these sensors in our brains called mirror neurons that pick up on the emotions of other people and mimic those feelings in our own body[1]. It's one of the key ways we connect, empathise and build emotional relationships with others.

Fish Feelings

This emotional contagion is my theory as to why we believed for so long that fish don't have feelings: because they don't have expressions on their faces. It's easy to see the pain in a dog's or a cow's eyes and instantly resonate with it, but fish don't use facial expressions to communicate, so there's nothing for our mirror neurons to pick up on. And so for many years before science caught up, we would happily gobble down the poor fishy, ignorant to the very real fact that the sentient being 100% suffered before landing on our dinner plate.

Here's how this emotional contagion works for vegans. If you're loving your plant-based cooking, feeling inspired for saving the planet, glowing with empowerment every time you ask for oat milk in your coffee, smiling when you wear your 'Friends, Not Food' T-shirt, or excited when they've got vegan cake at the buffet, then other people are picking up on those emotions, and something inside them is wanting what you're having. They might not even realise and will probably deny it—even to themselves if they're hardcore meat eaters—but the seed has been planted.

We owe it to the movement to do the best we can and to enjoy what we're doing. If leading the protest march to the gates of the chicken farm or being part of an Anonymous Cube of Truth protest in a busy shopping mall really lights you up, then go for it. If you take pleasure in cooking for others and sharing your creations, then do more of that. If you demonstrate your commitment by asking for vegan options in restaurants and walking out if they have none, then keep walking. Even if all you do is silently eat your mixed bean salad while subtly leave a magazine on the table, open at an interesting article on the plant-based lifestyle, then that's amazing too.

Remember, there's no such thing as perfect vegans. Animal products are in our roads, our money, our taxes, and also: we're humans, not robots. We have competing priorities and complicated social relationships. We have our mental health to consider, as well as the fact that habits take time to build and are easier to sustain over the long term when there's flexibility. There are also unconscious psychological processes, like consensus and confirmation bias, influencing us inside our own brains.

Holding ourselves and others to unobtainable standards of

Chapter 11: Be the Lighthouse

perfection will only make it harder and less inspiring for others to join the journey. Carnism already means that society is set up to work against us. The unexamined and hidden ideology of carnism, as Melanie Joy says, 'enables compassionate people to support cruel practices and to not even realise what they're doing.' We were most likely one of those people in the past—in your case, maybe even right up until you started this book—so we must remember to have compassion for others, too. People in our lives who haven't gone vegan yet aren't bad people—they are just humans doing the best they can with what they know and what they care about.

Sometimes the best thing we can do is just plant seeds. We know we can't change people by force. Did someone force *you* to go vegan? People can only change when inspired to do so internally, when the seed inside them becomes a fully grown garden and needs to burst out and express itself.

Everyone loves to be rewarded and recognised. With your partner, close friends, people at work—and even yourself—instead of nit-picking everything they're doing wrong, celebrate all the good steps they're taking. Appreciation begets more of the same. It's a foundation of behavioural psychology that learning is reinforced by rewards. When we receive a reward (and it can be as simple as an appreciative smile or some kind words), then we get a hit of dopamine and are encouraged to sustain the behaviour that gained us that reward[2].

Recently, I was talking with a friend at work about not being a perfect vegan. They were telling me how they were vegan for a year when they were working part-time, but that they went back to a normal diet when work got busy. I validated that. I reminded them that, as a human, they have different priorities at different times and assured them that they were doing the best they could. They kept saying, 'Yeah, but I could do more' or 'Hmmm—it's not really an excuse, is it?' I kept validating, and it ended with a self-inspired commitment to do more. It kind of seemed like I was using reverse psychology—although that wasn't my intention, I swear. I simply validated their experiences and appreciated the good they did.

As the proverb says, 'You catch more flies with honey than with vinegar.' (Not that we want to trap flies, nor do vegans use honey, but you get the metaphor.)

~

We're on a mission to save the world. And to do so, we need to give up animal products. It's not going to happen overnight, but it *will* get easier over time. Once that giant boulder gets over the tipping point, it'll begin to roll downhill and gather momentum along the way. We need collective action to set it in motion—we need as many people as possible being as vegan as they can be—and once it's in motion, it frees up other people to act as well. It makes plant-based the default option. And remember, human evolution designed us to take the easy option.

Luckily, this collective action started decades ago, and some cultures have been doing this for their whole existence. It's now easier than ever to be vegan. Every little thing you can do will help the cause and push that boulder along. Together, we can reduce animal suffering, reverse the effects of carbon emissions, grow back our forests, repopulate our biodiversity, save our coastlines from rising seas, replenish our oceans, and

Chapter 11: Be the Lighthouse

re-oxygenate our coral reefs. We can be a kinder world, with humans who support each other and cheer each other on.

It might sound like just a dreamy mission, but I know it's possible. Besides, I'd rather work towards a beautiful vision than give up our one and only home.

FINAL WORDS: Making a Difference

From a biological standpoint, humans can handle eating animals. In survival situations, like much of our ancestral past, we ate them alongside plants and survived long enough to reproduce. While there's nothing biologically wrong with eating animals, what's wrong is the *way* we do it. Animals in our modern agriculture are so far removed from their natural state, and so unhealthy themselves, that it becomes biologically unsafe to consume them. Farmed animals are mistreated and abused for the sake of supplying a falsely created demand, with no regard to how these practices are destroying our home planet, and, in our affluent Western society, we don't actually *need* to get our nutrients from animals.

Factory farming has taken over the world, and traditional farmers have been replaced by scientists with degrees in

Final Words: Making a Difference

agricultural production and consumer marketing, with a focus on increasing profits, lowering cost, and inflating our demand to sell more. The connection with the land, animals, and community is gone. The *humanity* is gone. While it's true that there are pockets of traditional farms scattered throughout the world, the majority of the world's meat comes from intensive factory farms with terrible conditions, pollution, and disease risk. The rest of the meat that comes from idyllic countryside pastures is using more land than we've got space for, and potentially releasing more methane. Our seafood either comes from lice- and pesticide-infected cramped pens that pollute the surrounding ocean, or from wild fishing that's dredging the ocean's carbon sinks faster than deforestation in the Amazon. We're endangering species through bycatch, and we're discarding billions of tonnes of plastics that clog up the Great Pacific Garbage Patch and the stomachs of fish we eat.

Importantly, we don't *need* animals for a balanced diet. Evidence from around the world, like in our Blue Zones, demonstrates that we can have a long, thriving, and productive life by eating mostly plants. Sure, some nutrients are more easily packaged in animals, but the same goes for other types of foods. Animal meats may be high in protein and iron, but they're missing many vital micronutrients like vitamin C and fibre. Our bodies evolved on varied diets, and our gut microbiome thrives better with a diverse array of plants compared to the three or four animal meats we rotate. There's no one superfood that contains all the nutrients we need to survive, but a well-planned plant-based diet can give us everything we need.

Even though we know this intellectually, it can take time to get it right. It takes time to adjust our tastebuds, to learn new recipes, to figure out how to cook good-tasting tofu, and to learn which lentils to use in each type of dish. I promise these are all skills you'll be happy to master! We might have to go through a long period of trial and error to work out which skincare and household products work for us. We can't expect to suddenly wake up the next day and have a fully stocked kitchen and bathroom cabinet; besides the cost of replacing all these items, it may also depend on product availability in your area, like my yoghurts.

Some people have thrown out their existing items to start fresh, and others keep using what they've got until it runs out. We all do what's right for us and we all make balanced choices to manage our competing priorities, which may incorporate a range of requirements like avoiding single-use plastic, supporting mental health, minimising harm to animals, and eating well while traveling for work. We may make different choices in different situations, and different choices from one day to the next. Changing our minds, making mistakes, not getting it perfect—these things make us human, not hypocrites.

You're *allowed* to be human. Remember, the perfect vegan doesn't exist, and neither does perfection in any other area of life. Long-term success in anything relies more on consistency than it does on perfection. Perfection leads to burnout (and it's *so* boring). The best way to support yourself and encourage others to join you is to believe that we're all doing our best,

Final Words: Making a Difference

and we'll inspire others simply by living well and enjoying the journey. It's a well-established fact that we get more of the behaviour we reward. Not only for others in your life, but for yourself too—celebrate the things done well, and have compassion for the mistakes and for the different journeys we're all on. Acknowledge and appreciate every little thing you do that's pointing you in the right direction.

The animal industry has a massive impact on the health of our planet, and a handful of people doing veganism really well isn't going to make a dent. The only thing that *will* make a dent in this and generate momentum is the vast majority of people reducing their demand for meat and other animal products. The momentum will carry the rest of the world, and then it will become normal and expected to eat mostly plants. It'll be easier to find plant-based food; animal by-products will dry up; and cosmetics will turn to cheaper, plant-based alternatives. And, thankfully, corporations won't have as much money for lobbying, leaving our nutrition to science (where it should have been delegated all along).

~

If this was easy, it would already be done. Most people agree that they don't want animals to suffer, *and* they want to avoid climate change, *and* they want to eat healthy whole foods. If plant-based was the default, nearly everyone would do it. Even though eating a plant-based diet and being as vegan as possible goes a long way to achieving all these goals, our modern world isn't set up to support this. We need as many of us as possible to continue pushing that boulder over the tipping point so that it becomes easier for all of us.

But there are forces working against us. Our internal psychology wants us to take the easy route, and it doesn't like change. We feel societal pressure to fit in and be 'normal'. Carnism is a self-perpetuating myth that keeps itself hidden. And because our world is a global ecosystem in which action in one place can generate far away effects on the other side of the planet, the environmental damage isn't always obvious in our own little corner. Just because we don't see the damage caused when we take a bite of a burger—the deforested rainforest, the freshwater used, the methane released—it doesn't mean that it's not happening.

I grew up in places where animal farming doesn't *look* like it's bad for the environment. Driving recently through country Victoria and southern New Zealand, all I could see on the vast green landscape were cows roaming free on the rolling hills, open-sided barns, and lots of trees. Idyllic. 'Perfect', even. I didn't see smog hanging over the hills, nor pillars of smoke billowing from barns, and there were no dirty, polluted rivers. It looked nice and peaceful and green. It looked normal.

Besides the fact that big factory farms and their polluted sludge pools are being kept well off main roads and intentionally out of site, the majority of a farm's destruction happens in other countries, like the ocean dead zones at the end of the river it sits by, or the deforestation used to produce feed crops in the Amazon. That's one reason why it's so hard for Westerners to make the switch, to connect the dots: we don't see it firsthand. We're not even the first to experience climate change effects like

Final Words: Making a Difference

the floods, landslides, and droughts in Bangladesh, northern Africa, and Spain. Everything just seems normal to us. But one day, it won't be. And by then it will be too late.

This isn't a slow burn that will happen in thousands or even hundreds of years. Climate change will happen in the next 30 to 80 years, not only affecting my own quality of life, but the next generation too. Our children will be living through it. Unlike our ancestors who didn't know the damage they were causing, our generation *knows*. We are ancestors of the future, and it's our job to make sure there's a future to remember us.

We have the opportunity *now* to do something about it. We have the science, and it's getting more and more clear with stronger studies in recent years. We can no longer bury our head in the sand and say that we don't know. And we can't pretend it's up to the government or corporations to change their ways. Policy change is too slow and too wimpy. The market responds to consumer demand, and it actually moves really fast. Our strongest hope for changing the animal agriculture industry is to reduce our demand. Fighting for government policy is worthy and necessary (so please don't stop), but it's faster, easier, and cheaper to vote with our wallet and change our diet. Nothing makes governments and corporations stand up and take notice more than dwindling profits.

Climate change and the mindset of carnism is like a disease on our planet, incubating. We need to do everything we can to make our Mother Earth well, before the disease takes hold fully and there's no turning back. We *will* reach a tipping point one way or another—either into continual feedback loops of rising sea temperatures and melting ice caps (that's the bad scenario) or into a majority plant-based diet across the world. This book is my contribution to the latter scenario, and I hope you'll join me, in any way that works for you. We've covered a myriad of ways right here in these pages, and it's my sincere hope that some of them have resonated.

~

We don't all need to be the sort of vegan who rams it down others' throats. 'Quiet activism' is just doing your thing and being happy about it. Once while on a flight, I asked the attendant if she had any vegan options, and it opened the door for her to ask me about being vegan. She'd always wanted to try it but thought it was too hard. She said that she could never give up chocolate, and I just happened to have some of the new vegan Lindt in my bag, so I gave her a piece to try. She ended by saying that she'd give it a go from there on out. Whether or not she did isn't in my control, but I know that I planted a seed.

Yes, our choices are ours entirely, and on their own have no impact on the global scale, but what we eat inspires others—at the very least to make them question and think. We're making a statement just by eating! You can save the world just by doing your bit without forcing anyone around you to change. That's quiet activism right there—and it works brilliantly.

If, like me, you just can't sit still because this is something you're so passionate about, consider adding your voice to the cause. It's natural to want to share what you're learning and care deeply about. You want to educate others and hope they'll

Final Words: Making a Difference

join you. It can also feel overwhelming and frustrating when you can see *so clearly* and others just don't seem to get it. But one thing I've learnt through experience, and witnessing others, is the power of keeping emotions in check. Easier said than done, I know, but angry attacks will only make people more defensive.

One of the vegans I interviewed for this book told me an example of her sister-in-law who was an extreme and angry vegan. Part of her pledge was to never sit at a table where animals were being served. This in itself is fine, but as a guest at a family wedding, she refused to sit at the family table, verbally abused other family members, and stood in a doorway glaring at them as they ate. My friend said that her vegetarian mother came the closest she'd ever come to eating meat just to spite this person. Anger and attacks—especially when people are eating—only get people's backs up, and can even cause peace-loving vegetarians to go the opposite way. It not only doesn't work for what's intended—it works *against* the cause. And nobody wants an angry, shouting activist in their face. There are much more effective (and friendlier) ways to teach others.

Being supportive, encouraging, curious, and polite is going to spread your message a lot further than being defensive, angry, and nit-picky. Seek first to understand where people are coming from, and what *their* competing priorities are. What are they trying to balance? Ask questions to figure out what they know, and check for permission before sharing some of your knowledge. Your knowledge will most likely contradict theirs, and if they haven't given you permission to share with them, their mind will be automatically closed and defensive.

The Imperfect Vegan

Remember to choose your timing as well—*not* while they're eating. (Again—sorry, Mum.)

If you want to get involved, check out the resources at the end of this book, where I've provided links to organisations that support vegan activism.

Whether you want to be an activist or just eat your plants in peace, and whether you've completely converted or are dabbling with something like Meat Free Mondays, thank you for your contribution to saving our planet. You are, without doubt, making more of a difference than you could possibly know.

~

Whatever we choose to do can be a challenge, but most of the time, I honestly do love being vegan. I love getting my meals first on the airplane. I love the variety of plants I eat and the rainbow of colours on my plate. I love exploring new recipes and being pleasantly surprised that they taste good (the number of times you serve yourself some kind of new vegan delight and self-congratulate your kitchen skills will astound you). I love cooking up a veggie-full lentil stew, or whipping up a quick and colourful buddha bowl, and I love how Phil enjoys them, too (even if he takes more than his fair share sometimes—but that's just further proof to me of how *good* this stuff is).

I love the feeling of aligning with my values when I ask for vegan products, or when I walk away from a restaurant that has no vegan options. It lines up with my internal compass, and I feel like (edit: I *know*) I'm doing the right thing. I know

Final Words: Making a Difference

that I'm making a difference and doing something good in the world. When I talk with others and share my food, I feel like I'm being inspiring and planting seeds that may one day change the world. I love talking about vegan stuff, having debates with people, and sharing facts and studies that counteract the beliefs we've been fed by the media. I loved researching and writing this book, and I absolutely love that you're reading it.

However, I won't lie: There are times when I wish I didn't know all this. Sometimes it feels like it's easier to just give up. Ignorance really *is* bliss, and there've been many occasions (and there'll be more, I'm sure) when I feel like just reverting back to mainstream and not caring. Midway through the book, I wrote this journal entry (unedited except for grammar):

It feels heavy. It feels like I'm the only one awake, and everyone around me is asleep, or blind. And if they are awake, they don't care. I feel like I'm carrying the weight of this problem for the whole world. Sometimes I think it would just be easier to not care. To continue living my life of abundance and consumerism. The world might get a little worse in my lifetime, but it probably won't be apocalyptic. I don't personally have kids or grandkids to worry about, so why don't I just enjoy my life and take as much as I can, and then when I'm dead, I won't care about the planet. Seems like that's what everyone else is doing. Why even write this book?

But it's not in my nature. I will never stop trying. I'm an action person, and I'm an influencer. If I see a better way, I will strive for it. And I will do my best to show others the light. I sound like a religious fanatic now. I get why religions went to war, if they felt their way was right and if they believed that they had to save everyone to save themselves. If they believed that people living a different way than them meant that they wouldn't get to heaven, then of course they would do everything they could to convince other people to change.

Is vegan a religion? Are we right? What's the worst that can happen if we convince the world to go vegan and we're wrong? Animals won't suffer anymore, although we may lose some species like the cows and chickens we've genetically bred. There'll be more space, land. But if we're right, and we do nothing, what's the worst then? Well, we might not be around to see it. We might be fighting for survival on high ground because our coastal cities have flooded and disrupted worldwide shipping routes, and the internet is gone because there's no electrical grid. So we won't even know what's happening in other parts of the world. We'll all be hunting and gathering and eating whatever animals and plants we can find then. Phil's looking forward to it. He calls it the zombie apocalypse, but climate, zombies, nuclear...whatever it'll be. He's ready to live wild and fight for survival. I reckon I'd tap out if it got to that. So maybe that's why he doesn't care about eating meat right now. He's confident he'll survive in a crisis, so why change now? Enjoy the luxuries of life while we've got them, and then enjoy the survival race later. Best of both worlds.

That was my actual journal entry—my in-the-moment thoughts while having a moment of panic. I still feel like this sometimes, but as I finish writing this book, I continue to believe that vegan is the right thing to do. It's certainly not the

Final Words: Making a Difference

only thing we need to do to save our planet, but I feel good knowing that I'm doing what I can.

A friend of mine at the gym has a tattoo that says, 'If you give less, I will give double.' I don't know exactly what it means to her, but to me it symbolises that we've got work to do. This shit needs to get done, and for those who choose to be slack about it, I'll step up and show them what's possible. I see it as a big eff you (ahem) to people who aren't pulling their weight. Enough is enough. If there are individuals around me who aren't supporting the plant, I'm the sort of person who will do what's needed for the sake of the bigger picture.

It may be hard sometimes, and I may not be perfect (happily imperfect, actually), but I can't go through life knowing the truth and not doing anything about it. Anything else I considered using my life for—business coaching, mental health counselling, owning a gym—all of this is secondary to ensuring that our planet is habitable so that future generations can follow their dreams without having to worry about survival. We are the ancestors of the future. I have to do my bit, even if my actions are inconsequential, and even if no one around me is doing anything.

But there *are* people out there doing something. There *are* people everywhere supporting this movement. Some are hardcore vegans who hate my message, some are curious onlookers asking questions. Some are people inventing yummy plant-based food, or doctors promoting the health benefits of veganism. There's animal liberation political parties, protestors who stay focused on the government change, and even family members who serve vegan dishes when I come to visit.

I mentioned at the start of this book that we're growing—and we are. We're coming to a tipping point where plant-based will become the default and where it'll be easier for everyone.

Until then, as imperfect vegans, we keep our head up, we hold compassion, we make conscious choices, we be the lighthouse. Why? Because we *are* making a difference.

Who saved the world?
No one did.
Yeah, but who saved the world?
Everyone did.

WHAT'S NEXT?

If you're inspired by what you've read here, I invite you to join me so we can celebrate each other for all the good we do.

Let's create a world that's plant-based by default, that encourages and supports all the progress along the journey.

Connect, find resources and receive support at:

catwhite.net/imperfectvegan

Plus, as a valued reader, you can grab a special bonus with food ideas and some of my favourite simple and nutritious recipes. Free!

ACKNOWLEDGEMENTS

Writing a book, and especially self-publishing, involves many people. Since I'm not the sort of person to whip something up with the help (or hindrance!) of AI and chuck it onto Amazon, I engaged professionals to help with every step of the process. (And, just for the avoidance of doubt, these *are* all my words—no ChatGPT made its way into this book.)

My first sentiments of gratitude go to my editor Rob Peace, because finding him became the cornerstone of this entire project. He not only helped me finesse my words and polish the manuscript, but he also made me feel so validated as a writer. He brought a unique skill of being able to inject wit, candour, and CERT (he knows what that means) where it was needed while still retaining my original voice. He also provided invaluable input on cover design, formatting ideas, fact checking, and even my TEDx speech.

After the editing process, Sophia Munnik meticulously pulled out the references from the document and built the reference list, allowing me to create the very helpful online version that anyone

Acknowledgements

can access to do their own research. Shehzad Saleem adapted all images and graphs into black and white, and simplified them to make them suitable for smaller print. Tonia Nazzaro then worked her formatting and typesetting magic on converting a Word document into the readable and professional-looking paperback or ebook you're holding in your hands. For the cover, the talented Steph Webber worked tirelessly on creating the perfect design and dealt with my many iterations and midnight ideas, but we finally landed on something we love, and I hope that you love it, too.

Once the book was all pulled together, my team of proof-readers included friends and family who went through it with a fine-toothed comb to find the punctuation and grammar errors that myself and Rob would have undoubtedly missed after spending so much time reading the same lines over and over. Thanks Dad, Jos, Kaylee and Suzanne. And to Liz and JD from Weekend Publisher, a huge thank you for the short course and ongoing support on marketing and publishing for authors. From these incredible humans, I learnt how to make this book available for sale, discoverable in search results, and attractive to readers, meaning that it can reach more people and have an even bigger impact on the world.

Creating the content of the book took a village as well.

Thanks to researchers, academics, filmmakers, and other vegan educators and activists who responded to my requests for information, references, and clarification. Your willingness to respond to an (as-yet) unknown author demonstrates your passion for supporting the cause and helping to educate the world. A special shout out goes to Kiah, Megan, and the team at Plant Nutrition and Wellness, who spent time reviewing the nutrition sections of the book to make sure that what I'm sharing with you is accurate and healthy.

The Imperfect Vegan

As a university student, I'm incredibly grateful that I have free access to libraries and research databases around the world. Many of the documents and studies I reference throughout the book have come from journals that require a paid subscription, but as a student, I receive free access through my institution. This has saved me time and money, and it's given me access to top-quality research.

Even more valuable than academic works have been the countless conversations with real people: vegans, imperfect vegans, and mainstream dieters; slaughterhouse workers and farm owners; and anyone who would listen, really. Special thanks to Belinda for not only planting the seed that inspired this book, but also for our long chats about building a vegan world. Thank you to Alyse, Arriel, Ashleigh, Belinda, Brett, Clark, Connie, David, Hanna, Jacinta, James, Jasmin, Josh, Louise, Luke, Maddy, Mat, Rachel, Shea, Tamsin, Tom, Tracey, and many more who inspired me with your stories, experiences, firsthand knowledge, and advice and transition tips for others.

Most all, thank you to Phil for being my sturdy tree. You patiently accept that I spend most of my time working on, thinking of, or talking about my book. But more than just listening to my ramblings, you ask me questions to help clarify my thinking, share your own insights, and 'talk me up' to other people. I truly appreciate how you pull me away from the computer when I'm getting stressed, and how your support extends to both dragging me to the gym and keeping me in a constant supply of vegan chocolate. Most of all, I love and appreciate you for supporting me in following my passions, even though you're not on the same path (yet!). I love us.

HELPFUL RESOURCES

Books

There are plenty of amazing books covering all aspects of the vegan lifestyle, but rather than providing you with a library, here are just some of my favourites:

Vegan Propaganda, **Ed Winters**
Ed is really good at the 'moral consideration' argument for why we shouldn't eat animals, something that I don't explore in depth in this book.
Another excellent resource of Ed's, his free e-book *30 Non-Vegan Excuses and How to Respond to Them* can be accessed directly here: https://www.all-creatures.org/articles2/act-earthling-ed.pdf

Why We Love Dogs, Eat Pigs, and Wear Cows, **Melanie Joy**
This delves into the psychology of our food choices, and introduces the concept of 'carnism,' which was the topic of Melanie Joy's PHD thesis. This is the book that woke me up.

The Proof Is in the Plants, **Simon Hill**
This book focuses on the health aspect of a plant-based diet, and I

love how real science is explained in easy-to-understand language.

***How to Argue With Vegans*, Benny Malone**
This is a book I picked up on a whim, but it actually had really insightful chapters on the types of language and patterns people use when we argue (or debate or converse), and it explores how to respond in each type of situation. I especially found it useful to know when to walk away!

***Slaughterhouse*, Gail Eisnitz**
A shocking exposé into the US slaughterhouse culture by an investigative journalist, covering not only animal abuse but also food safety and working conditions.

***We Are the Weather*, Jonathan Safran Foer**
Ultimately, this is a book about how our food choices impact our weather, but it's very cleverly written and full of seemingly unrelated but incredibly interesting stories that eventually come together to make his point. It also contains one of the simplest explanations of climate change I've come across.

***The Joyful Vegan*, Colleen Patrick-Goudreau**
Starting with the assumption that the reader is already on a vegan journey, this book focuses on navigating the social and cultural pressures of choosing to be vegan in a carnist world, and it helps us stay the course—joyfully.

Documentaries

Cowspiracy (2014)
https://www.cowspiracy.com
An expose of the damaging impacts of the animal agriculture industries on our environment.

Helpful Resources

Seaspiracy (2021)
https://www.seaspiracy.org
Like Cowspiracy, but focusing on the fishing industries.

Eating Our Way to Extinction (2021)
https://www.eating2extinction.com
Similar to Cowspiracy, but updated with the latest science. It contains excellent visual representations of statistics, so it's really clear to understand.

Forks over Knives (2011)
https://www.forksoverknives.com
One of the original plant-based advocates, this focuses on the health aspects of eating plant-based whole foods.

Dominion (2018)
https://www.dominionmovement.com/watch
An exposé of the Australian animal agriculture conditions. It's definitely not #*onlyinamerica*.

Land of Hope and Glory (2017)
https://www.landofhopeandglory.org
Produced by Earthling Ed's animal rights group, Surge, this film shows the truth about the UK animal industries.

Food

Plant Nutrition and Wellness
https://www.plantnutritionwellness.com
This is a small group of plant-based dietitians who specialise in helping people transition and adapt to a plant-based way of eating.

They're based in Brisbane, Queensland, but they can work with worldwide clients due to the magic of the internet. (Even though I'm Brisbane-based, all my sessions were virtual.)

Some of my favourite recipe websites for vegan inspiration:
Love and Lemons: https://www.loveandlemons.com
Cookie and Kate: https://cookieandkate.com
Minimalist Baker: https://minimalistbaker.com (not 100% vegan, but they have an incredible vegan recipe list)

Education

Healthline
https://www.healthline.com
A great resource for evidence-based research, generally unbiased, and they link to sources.

Farm Transparency Project
https://www.farmtransparency.org
An interactive map of Australia showing all farms, slaughterhouses, and other forms of animal exploitation. It includes documents, news, and activism campaigns.

Counterglow
https://www.counterglow.org
Similar to Farm Transparency, but for the US.

Our World in Data
https://ourworldindata.org
A global charity that focuses on translating data into visual representations to highlight the important issues of our world.

Helpful Resources

The Vegan Calculator
http://thevegancalculator.com/#calculator
A fun calculator to show how much water, animal lives, carbon, etc. that you've saved based on how long you've been vegan.

Carbon Brief
https://interactive.carbonbrief.org/what-is-the-climate-impact-of-eating-meat-and-dairy
A very detailed but easy-to-read report on our carbon emissions from meat and dairy.

Advocacy, Activism & Support Groups

We The Free
https://www.activism.wtf
Campaigns with non-violent street and online activism.

In Defense of Animals
https://www.idausa.org/campaign/sustainable-activism/animal-activist-helpline
An activist support line. Free counselling for dealing with the emotional ups and downs of this work.

VegFund
https://vegfund.org
Empowering global animal rights activism, with financial grants for advocacy and action.

Plant Based Treaty
https://plantbasedtreaty.org
As a companion to the Paris Agreement, this a worldwide treaty

aiming to halt the destruction of our ecosystem by animal agriculture, and to restore our natural environment. You can endorse as an individual or a business, or petition your local councillors to sign as a city.

The Vreedom Quest
https://www.thevreedomquest.com
An online community with webinars and courses to inspire vegan changemakers. Its ambitious mission is to create a 50% vegan world by 2030.

REFERENCES

For your ease of access, all resources and references are listed and clickable online at catwhite.net/imperfectvegan-references.

Introduction
1. Steinfeld, H., Gerber, P., Wassenaar, T.D., et al. (2006). Livestock's Long Shadow: Environmental Issues and Options. https://www.fao.org/3/a0701e/a0701e.pdf
2. UN. (n.d.). Goal 13: Take Urgent Action to Combat Climate Change and Its Impacts. https://www.un.org/sustainabledevelopment/climate-change/
3. Pearce, R. & Huasfather, Z. (2018). Mapped: How Every Part of the World Has Warmed – and Could Continue to Warm. https://www.carbonbrief.org/mapped-how-every-part-of-the-world-has-warmed-and-could-continue-to-warm/
4. NASA Earth Observatory. (2020). Global Temperatures. https://earthobservatory.nasa.gov/world-of-change/global-temperatures
5. Lindsey, R. & Dahlman, L. (2023). Climate Change: Global Temperature. http://www.climate.gov/news-features/understanding-climate/climate-change-global-temperature
6. FAO. (n.d.). Key Facts and Findings. https://www.fao.org/news/story/en/item/197623/icode/
7. Climate Nexus. (2016). Animal Agriculture's Impact on Climate Change. https://climatenexus.org/climate-issues/food/animal-agricultures-impact-on-climate-change/
8. UN News. (2006). Rearing Cattle Produces More Greenhouse Gases than Driving Cars, UN Report Warns. https://news.un.org/en/story/2006/11/201222-rearing-cattle-produces-more-greenhouse-gases-

driving-cars-un-report-warns
9. WWF. (2018). What Are the Biggest Drivers of Tropical Deforestation? https://www.worldwildlife.org/magazine/issues/summer-2018/articles/what-are-the-biggest-drivers-of-tropical-deforestation
10. UNEP. (2021). Our Global Food System Is the Primary Driver of Biodiversity Loss. http://www.unep.org/news-and-stories/press-release/our-global-food-system-primary-driver-biodiversity-loss
11. Kubiak, L. (2019). Marine Biodiversity in Dangerous Decline, Finds New Report. https://www.nrdc.org/bio/lauren-kubiak/marine-biodiversity-dangerous-decline-finds-new-report
12. National Geographic. (2022). Dead Zone. https://education.nationalgeographic.org/resource/dead-zone
13. Denchak, M. (2023). Water Pollution Definition - Types, Causes, Effects. https://www.nrdc.org/stories/water-pollution-everything-you-need-know
14. Egger, M. (2022). Where Is Plastic in the Great Pacific Garbage Patch From? https://theoceancleanup.com/updates/the-other-source-where-does-plastic-in-the-great-pacific-garbage-patch-come-from/
15. FAO. (2019). Water Use in Livestock Production Systems and Supply Chains- Guidelines for Assessment: Version 1. https://www.fao.org/3/ca5685en/ca5685en.pdf
16. Heinke, J., Lannerstad, M., Gerten, D., et al. (2020). Water Use in Global Livestock Production—Opportunities and Constraints for Increasing Water Productivity. https://onlinelibrary.wiley.com/doi/abs/10.1029/2019WR026995
17. Ritchie, H. (2017). How Much of the World's Land Would We Need in Order to Feed the Global Population with the Average Diet of a given Country? https://ourworldindata.org/agricultural-land-by-global-diets
18. Human Rights Watch (Organization). (2004). Blood, Sweat, and Fear: Workers' Rights in U.s. Meat and Poultry Plants. https://www.fao.org/3/a0701e/a0701e.pdf
19. Hayek, M.N. (2022). The Infectious Disease Trap of Animal Agriculture. https://www.science.org/doi/10.1126/sciadv.add6681
20. PCRM. (2021). U.S. Meat and Dairy Companies Spend Millions Lobbying Against Climate Legislation. https://www.pcrm.org/news/blog/us-meat-and-dairy-companies-spend-millions-lobbying-against-climate-legislation
21. The Vegan Society. (n.d.). Definition of Veganism. https://www.vegansociety.com/go-vegan/definition-veganism
22. The Vegan Web Designer. (n.d.). The Vegan Calculator. https://www.thevegancalculator.com
23. Weber, C.L. & Matthews, H.S. (2008). Food-Miles and the Relative Climate Impacts of Food Choices in the United States. https://doi.org/10.1021/

References

es702969f

24. Ridler, G. (2022). "Record Year" for Investment into Meat Alternatives. https://www.foodmanufacture.co.uk/Article/2022/03/03/Record-year-for-investment-into-meat-alternatives
25. Coyne, A. (2023). Eyeing Alternatives – Meat Companies with Stakes in Meat-Free and Cell-Based Meat. https://www.just-food.com/features/eyeing-alternatives-meat-companies-with-stakes-in-meat-free-and-cell-based-meat/
26. Bottinelli, S. (2022). Celebrities Investing in Plant-Based Food Companies. https://foodmatterslive.com/gallery/tech-moguls-sports-personalities-and-celebrities-investing-in-plant-based-food-companies/
27. Torrella, K. (2023). Were the Impossible and Beyond Burgers a Fad, or Is Plant-Based Meat Here to Stay? https://www.vox.com/future-perfect/2023/4/17/23682232/impossible-beyond-plant-based-meat-sales
28. Speciality Food. (2023). Plant-Based Growth Continues. https://www.specialtyfood.com/news/article/plant-based-growth-continues/
29. Minassian, L. (2022). Why the Global Rise in Vegan and Plant-Based Eating Is No Fad (30x Increase in US Vegans + Other Astounding Vegan Stats). https://foodrevolution.org/blog/vegan-statistics-global/
30. Ignaszewski, E. & Pierece, B. (2021). Retail Sales Data: Plant-Based Meat, Eggs, Dairy. https://gfi.org/marketresearch/
31. Rabb, M. (2022). Plant-Based Menu Items Spiked Nearly 3,000 Percent Since 2018. https://thebeet.com/plant-based-menu-options-study/
32. Ethical Elephant. (2021). 9 Popular Beauty Brands Go 100% Vegan Because of Us! https://ethicalelephant.com/beauty-brands-go-vegan/
33. NYC Public Schools. (n.d.). Plant-Powered Meals. https://www.schools.nyc.gov/school-life/food/school-meals/plant-powered
34. NYC Health + Hospitals. (2023). NYC Health + Hospitals Now Serving Plant-Based Meals as Primary Dinner Option for Inpatients At All of Its 11 Public Hospitals. https://www.nychealthandhospitals.org/pressrelease/nyc-health-hospitals-now-serving-plant-based-meals-as-primary-dinner-option-for-inpatients-at-all-of-its-11-public-hospitals/
35. Starostinetskaya, A. (2019). Amsterdam Pledges to Serve Meatless Meals at Government Meetings. https://vegnews.com/2019/5/amsterdam-pledges-to-serve-meatless-meals-at-government-meetings
36. Vegconomist. (2023). Taiwan Passes Climate Bill Mandating the Promotion of Plant-Based Foods. https://vegconomist.com/politics-law/taiwan-climate-bill-promotion-plant-based-foods/
37. Vegans Baby. (2023). Vegan Dining Month. https://vegansbaby.com/vegan-dining-month/
38. Lingenfelter, J. (2023). A Record Number of People Worldwide Participate in Veganuary 2023. https://veganuary.com/en-us/record-number-of-people-

worldwide-participate-in-veganuary-2023/
39. Poinski, M. (2022). Consumer Awareness of Food's Environmental Impact Is Slowly Growing. https://www.fooddive.com/news/kearney-report-food-environmental-impacts-consumers/622354/

Chapter 1

1. Beard, T. (2021). The Year Earth Changed. https://www.imdb.com/title/tt14372240/
2. Lecchini, D., Brooker, R.M., Waqalevu, V., et al. (2021). Effects of COVID-19 Pandemic Restrictions on Coral Reef Fishes at Eco-Tourism Sites in Bora-Bora, French Polynesia. https://linkinghub.elsevier.com/retrieve/pii/S0141113621002075
3. Tomlinson, H. (2020). Himalayas Come into View as Empty Roads Let Smog Clear. https://www.thetimes.co.uk/article/himalayas-come-into-view-as-empty-roads-let-smog-clear-rgdlsmqks
4. Struck, D. (n.d.). How the "Global Cooling" Story Came to Be. https://www.scientificamerican.com/article/how-the-global-cooling-story-came-to-be/
5. Bradford Telegraph and Argus. (2016). 42 PICTURES: Bradford Wakes up to Unseasonal Covering of Late April Snow. https://www.thetelegraphandargus.co.uk/news/14460881.42-pictures-bradford-wakes-up-to-unseasonal-covering-of-late-april-snow/
6. Phys Org. (2021). Moscow Melts in Historic June Heat Wave. https://phys.org/news/2021-06-moscow-battered-historic-june.html
7. Searle, J. (2010). Aussie Flood Zone Bigger than France and Germany Combined. https://www.nbcnews.com/id/wbna40858188
8. Ritchie, E.J. (2018). Exactly How Much Has the Earth Warmed? And Does It Matter? https://www.forbes.com/sites/uhenergy/2018/09/07/exactly-how-much-has-the-earth-warmed-and-does-it-matter/
9. UCAR. (2022). Why Earth Is Warming | Center for Science Education. https://scied.ucar.edu/learning-zone/how-climate-works/why-earth-warming
10. Buis, A. (2019). A Degree of Concern: Why Global Temperatures Matter. https://climate.nasa.gov/news/2865/a-degree-of-concern-why-global-temperatures-matter
11. Roberts, D. (2018). This Graphic Explains Why 2 Degrees of Global Warming Will Be Way Worse than 1.5. https://www.vox.com/energy-and-environment/2018/1/19/16908402/global-warming-2-degrees-climate-change
12. Lieberman, B. (2021). 1.5 or 2 Degrees Celsius of Additional Global Warming: Does It Make a Difference? http://yaleclimateconnections.org/2021/08/1-5-or-2-degrees-celsius-of-additional-global-warming-does-

References

it-make-a-difference/
13. WWF. (2018). Wildlife in a Warming World: The Effects of Climate Change on Biodiversity in WWF's Priority Places. https://files.worldwildlife.org/wwfcmsprod/files/Publication/file/558gtvwcut_WWF___Wildlife_in_a_Warming_World___2018_FINAL.pdf?_ga=2.120209547.282538411.1676761616-1278369021.1676320638
14. Xu, C., Kohler, T.A., Lenton, T.M., et al. (2020). Future of the Human Climate Niche. https://pnas.org/doi/full/10.1073/pnas.1910114117
15. IPCC. (2018). Infographic: The Difference in Projected Climate Impacts between 1.5°C and 2°C of Warming. https://www.climatecouncil.org.au/wp-content/uploads/2021/04/Infographic-page-35-scaled.jpg
16. Healthy Human Life. (2022). Why Are Coral Reefs Important for the Planet? https://healthyhumanlife.com/blogs/news/why-are-coral-reefs-important
17. Editors of EarthSky. (2015). How Much Do Oceans Add to World's Oxygen? https://earthsky.org/earth/how-much-do-oceans-add-to-worlds-oxygen/
18. Pester, P. (2021). When Did Scientists First Warn Humanity about Climate Change? https://www.livescience.com/humans-first-warned-about-climate-change
19. UNFCCC. (2023). The Paris Agreement: What Is the Paris Agreement? https://unfccc.int/process-and-meetings/the-paris-agreement
20. World Bank. (2022). Key Highlights: Country Climate and Development Report for Bangladesh. https://www.worldbank.org/en/news/feature/2022/10/31/key-highlights-country-climate-and-development-report-for-bangladesh
21. WMO. (2022). State of Climate in Africa Highlights Water Stress and Hazards. https://public.wmo.int/en/media/press-release/state-of-climate-africa-highlights-water-stress-and-hazards
22. Pettigrew, S. (2020). Spanish Climate Migrants Strongly Correlated with Climate Justice. https://www.climatescorecard.org/2020/09/spanish-climate-migrants-strongly-correlated-with-climate-justice/
23. Carbon Brief Staff. (2021). In-Depth Q&A: The IPCC's Sixth Assessment Report on Climate Science. https://www.carbonbrief.org/in-depth-qa-the-ipccs-sixth-assessment-report-on-climate-science/
24. Forster, P., Rosen, D., Lamboll, R., et al. (2022). What the Tiny Remaining 1.5C Carbon Budget Means for Climate Policy. https://www.carbonbrief.org/guest-post-what-the-tiny-remaining-1-5c-carbon-budget-means-for-climate-policy/
25. Foer, J.S. (2019). We Are the Weather: Saving the Planet Begins at Breakfast. https://www.amazon.com.au/We-Are-Weather-Saving-Breakfast/

dp/0374280002
26. Ritchie, H., Roser, M., & Rosado, P. (2020). CO_2 and Greenhouse Gas Emissions. https://ourworldindata.org/emissions-by-sector
27. Berardelli, J. & Niemczyk, K. (2021). The Great Dying: Earth's Largest-Ever Mass Extinction Is a Warning for Humanity. https://www.cbsnews.com/news/great-dying-permian-triassic-extinction-event-warning-humanity/
28. Steinfeld, H., Gerber, P., Wassenaar, T.D., et al. (2006). Livestock's Long Shadow: Environmental Issues and Options. https://www.fao.org/3/a0701e/a0701e.pdf
29. Goodland, R. & Anhang, J. (2009). Livestock and Climate Change. https://awellfedworld.org/wp-content/uploads/Livestock-Climate-Change-Anhang-Goodland.pdf
30. Carus, F. (2010). UN Urges Global Move to Meat and Dairy-Free Diet. https://www.theguardian.com/environment/2010/jun/02/un-report-meat-free-diet
31. Frischmann, C. (2018). 100 Solutions to Reverse Global Warming. https://www.ted.com/talks/chad_frischmann_100_solutions_to_reverse_global_warming
32. Wynes, S. & Nicholas, K.A. (2017). The Climate Mitigation Gap: Education and Government Recommendations Miss the Most Effective Individual Actions. https://iopscience.iop.org/article/10.1088/1748-9326/aa7541
33. Lazard, O. (2022). The Blind Spots of the Green Energy Transition. https://www.ted.com/talks/olivia_lazard_the_blind_spots_of_the_green_energy_transition
34. Center for Sustainable Systems. (2022). Carbon Footprint Factsheet. https://css.umich.edu/publications/factsheets/sustainability-indicators/carbon-footprint-factsheet
35. Scarborough, P., Appleby, P.N., Mizdrak, A., et al. (2014). Dietary Greenhouse Gas Emissions of Meat-Eaters, Fish-Eaters, Vegetarians and Vegans in the UK. https://doi.org/10.1007/s10584-014-1169-1
36. Loken, B. & WWF. (2020). Bending the Curve: The Restorative Power of Planet-Based Diets. https://wwfeu.awsassets.panda.org/downloads/bending_the_curve__the_restorative_power_of_planet_based_diets_full_report_final_pdf.pdf
37. Ritchie, H. (2021). If the World Adopted a Plant-Based Diet We Would Reduce Global Agricultural Land Use from 4 to 1 Billion Hectares. https://ourworldindata.org/land-use-diets
38. Ritchie, H. & Roser, M. (2013). Land Use. https://ourworldindata.org/land-use
39. Sigler, J., Videle, J., Perry, C., et al. (2022). Animal-Based Agriculture Vs. Plant-Based Agriculture. A Multi-Product Data Comparison. https://

References

humaneherald.files.wordpress.com/2017/12/animal-vs-plant-based-agriculture.pdf

40. Poore, J. & Nemecek, T. (2018). Land Use per 100 Grams of Protein: Land Use Is Measured in Meters Squared (M^2) per 100 Grams of Protein across Various Food Products. https://ourworldindata.org/grapher/land-use-protein-poore
41. ARWEC. (2020). Water Facts - Worldwide Water Supply. https://www.usbr.gov/mp/arwec/water-facts-ww-water-sup.html
42. FAO. (2019). Water Use in Livestock Production Systems and Supply Chains- Guidelines for Assessment: Version 1. https://www.fao.org/3/ca5685en/ca5685en.pdf
43. Mekonnen, M.M. & Hoekstra, A.Y. (2012). A Global Assessment of the Water Footprint of Farm Animal Products. https://doi.org/10.1007/s10021-011-9517-8
44. Water Footprint Network. (2023). Do You Know How Much Water Was Used to Grow Your Food and to Produce Your Clothes and the Things You Buy? https://www.waterfootprint.org/time-for-action/what-can-consumers-do/
45. Ritchie, H. & Roser, M. (2017). Water Use and Stress. https://ourworldindata.org/water-use-stress
46. Chai, B.C., van der Voort, J.R., Grofelnik, K., et al. (2019). Which Diet Has the Least Environmental Impact on Our Planet? A Systematic Review of Vegan, Vegetarian and Omnivorous Diets. https://www.mdpi.com/2071-1050/11/15/4110
47. Poore, J. & Nemecek, T. (2018). Reducing Food's Environmental Impacts through Producers and Consumers. https://www.science.org/doi/10.1126/science.aaq0216
48. Heinke, J., Lannerstad, M., Gerten, D., et al. (2020). Water Use in Global Livestock Production—Opportunities and Constraints for Increasing Water Productivity. https://onlinelibrary.wiley.com/doi/abs/10.1029/2019WR026995
49. UNDESA. (2015). International Decade for Action "Water for Life" 2005-2015. Focus Areas: Water Scarcity. https://www.un.org/waterforlifedecade/scarcity.shtml
50. WHO. (2022). Drinking-Water. https://www.who.int/news-room/factsheets/detail/drinking-water
51. Brockway, O. & Brockway, L. (2022). Eating Our Way To Extinction | The Documentary. https://www.eating2extinction.com/
52. Vstats. (2023). Update: Animal Agriculture Drives 79% of Deforestation in Australia. https://vstats.substack.com/p/update-animal-agriculture-drives?mibextid=Zxz2cZ

53. Carrington, D. (2021). Amazon Rainforest Now Emitting More CO_2 than It Absorbs. https://www.theguardian.com/environment/2021/jul/14/amazon-rainforest-now-emitting-more-co2-than-it-absorbs
54. Pendrill, F., Persson, U.M., Godar, J., et al. (2019). Deforestation Displaced: Trade in Forest-Risk Commodities and the Prospects for a Global Forest Transition. https://dx.doi.org/10.1088/1748-9326/ab0d41
55. Ritchie, H. & Roser, M. (2021). Forests and Deforestation. https://ourworldindata.org/soy
56. NOAA. (n.d.). How Much Oxygen Comes from the Ocean? https://oceanservice.noaa.gov/facts/ocean-oxygen.html
57. NOAA. (2022). Quantifying the Ocean Carbon Sink. https://www.ncei.noaa.gov/news/quantifying-ocean-carbon-sink
58. Communications and Publishing. (2016). What a Drag: The Global Impact of Bottom Trawling | U.S. Geological Survey. https://www.usgs.gov/news/national-news-release/what-drag-global-impact-bottom-trawling
59. Hurlimann, S. (2019). How Kelp Naturally Combats Global Climate Change. https://sitn.hms.harvard.edu/flash/2019/how-kelp-naturally-combats-global-climate-change/
60. Davies, R.W.D., Cripps, S.J., Nickson, A., et al. (2009). Defining and Estimating Global Marine Fisheries Bycatch. https://assets.wwf.org.uk/downloads/bycatch_paper.pdf
61. Lindwall, C. (2022). Guide: Industrial Agricultural Pollution 101. https://www.nrdc.org/stories/industrial-agricultural-pollution-101
62. Scott, K. (2022). We Have International Laws to Stop Plastic Pollution from Fishing Vessels Now. Why Are We Not Enforcing Them? http://theconversation.com/we-have-international-laws-to-stop-plastic-pollution-from-fishing-vessels-now-why-are-we-not-enforcing-them-185951
63. Lebreton, L., Royer, S.-J., Peytavin, A., et al. (2022). Industrialised Fishing Nations Largely Contribute to Floating Plastic Pollution in the North Pacific Subtropical Gyre. https://www.nature.com/articles/s41598-022-16529-0
64. Climate Science. (2022). Fish Farming: Is Eating Fish Sustainable? https://climatescience.org/advanced-food-fishing-aquaculture
65. Martin, J. (2022). Scottish Salmon's Unsustainable Appetite – Who Benefits? https://feedbackglobal.org/scottish-salmons-unsustainable-appetite-who-benefits/
66. CTVC Team. (2021). Turning the Tide on Sustainable Seafood. https://www.ctvc.co/turning-the-tide-on-sustainable-seafood/
67. Frantz, D. & Collins, C. (2022). 3 Reasons to Avoid Farmed Salmon. https://time.com/6199237/is-farmed-salmon-healthy-sustainable/
68. Choudhury, A., Lepine, C., & Good, C. (2023). Methane and Hydrogen Sulfide Production from the Anaerobic Digestion of Fish Sludge from

References

Recirculating Aquaculture Systems: Effect of Varying Initial Solid Concentrations. https://www.mdpi.com/2311-5637/9/2/94
69. Humphreys, A.M., Govaerts, R., Ficinski, S.Z., et al. (2019). Global Dataset Shows Geography and Life Form Predict Modern Plant Extinction and Rediscovery. https://www.nature.com/articles/s41559-019-0906-2
70. IPBES. (2019). Summary for Policymakers of the Global Assessment Report on Biodiversity and Ecosystem Services. https://www.ipbes.net/sites/default/files/inline/files/ipbes_global_assessment_report_summary_for_policymakers.pdf
71. FAO. (2022). The State of World Fisheries and Aquaculture 2022. Towards Blue Transformation. https://www.fao.org/3/cc0461en/cc0461en.pdf
72. Stanescu, V. (2019). "Cowgate": Meat Eating and Climate Change Denial. *Climate Change Denial and Public Relations*. https://www.taylorfrancis.com/chapters/oa-edit/10.4324/9781351121798-11/cowgate-vasile-stanescu
73. Heller, M. (2015). Greenhouse Gas Emission Estimates of U.S. Dietary Choices and Food Loss. https://onlinelibrary.wiley.com/doi/pdfdirect/10.1111/jiec.12174

Chapter 2

1. Anderson, K. & Kuhn, K. (2014). COWSPIRACY: The Sustainability Secret. https://www.cowspiracy.com/
2. ALDF. (2015). Customary Cruelty in the Farm Industry: When Animal Abuse Is Legal. https://aldf.org/article/customary-cruelty-in-the-farm-industry-when-animal-abuse-is-legal/
3. AWI. (2018). Legal Protections for Animals on Farms. https://awionline.org/awi-quarterly/fall-2018
4. LCA. (2017). Legalized Cruelty: 10 Shocking Practices Directly from Animal Agriculture Policy. https://www.lcanimal.org/index.php/blog/entry/legalized-cruelty-10-shocking-practices-directly-from-animal-agriculture-policy
5. Farm Transparency Project. (2015). Pig Truth. https://www.farmtransparency.org/videos?id=0f06b4256b
6. Brennan, C. (2015). Landscaper Sentenced to Year in Prison for Running over Nine Ducklings. https://www.dailymail.co.uk/news/article-3175583/Landscaper-sentenced-year-prison-intentionally-running-nine-ducklings-laughing-horrified-family-feeding-bread.html
7. RSPCA. (2021). What Happens with Male Chicks in the Egg Industry? https://kb.rspca.org.au/knowledge-base/what-happens-with-male-chicks-in-the-egg-industry/
8. Farm Transparency Project. (2020). Age of Animals Slaughtered. https://www.farmtransparency.org/kb/food/abattoirs/age-animals-slaughtered

9. Turner, J., Garcés, L., & Smith, W. (2015). The Welfare of Broiler Chickens in the European Union. https://www.ciwf.org.uk/research/species-meat-chickens/the-welfare-of-broiler-chickens-in-the-european-union/
10. Charbeneau, D. (2019). The Number of Chickens Who Die Before Reaching the Kill Blade. https://animalequality.org/blog/2019/11/07/the-shocking-number-of-chickens-who-die-before-reaching-the-kill-blade/
11. Charbeneau, D. (2019). A Chicken's Last Day Revealed by Undercover Investigator. https://animalequality.org/blog/2019/12/19/what-one-undercover-investigator-revealed-about-a-chickens-last-day/
12. PETA. (2010). The Pork Industry. https://www.peta.org/issues/animals-used-for-food/factory-farming/pigs/pork-industry/
13. Anthis, K. & Anthis, J.R. (2019). Global Farmed & Factory Farmed Animals Estimates. https://sentienceinstitute.org/global-animal-farming-estimates
14. Anthis, J.R. (2019). US Factory Farming Estimates. https://sentienceinstitute.org/us-factory-farming-estimates
15. Kirby, M. (2013). Factory Farming Masks Meat's True Costs. https://www.abc.net.au/news/2013-06-21/kirby-modern-meat/4770226
16. Marinet Limited. (2021). The Scale of Intensive Indoor Livestock Farming in the United Kingdom, and the Impact of Its Related Sewage Disposal Regime upon Water Quality in Rivers. https://committees.parliament.uk/writtenevidence/23622/pdf/
17. Corselo. (2018). Archive: Small and Large Farms in the EU - Statistics from the Farm Structure Survey. https://ec.europa.eu/eurostat/statistics-explained/index.php?title=Archive:Small_and_large_farms_in_the_EU_-_statistics_from_the_farm_structure_survey
18. Klemperer, J. (2018). Why Slaughterhouse "Line Speeds" Matter. https://foodprint.org/blog/why-slaughterhouse-line-speeds-matter/
19. Warrick, J. (2001). "They Die Piece by Piece." https://www.washingtonpost.com/archive/politics/2001/04/10/they-die-piece-by-piece/f172dd3c-0383-49f8-b6d8-347e04b68da1/
20. de Haas, Y. (2013). Preventing Tail Biting in Pigs. https://www.wur.nl/en/dossiers/file/preventing-tail-biting-in-pigs.htm
21. O'Keefe, J. (2022). The Inhumane Psychological Treatment of Factory Farmed Animals. https://ffacoalition.org/articles/the-inhumane-psychological-treatment-of-factory-farmed-animals/
22. Jacobs, B. (2020). The Neural Cruelty of Captivity: Keeping Large Mammals in Zoos and Aquariums Damages Their Brains. http://theconversation.com/the-neural-cruelty-of-captivity-keeping-large-mammals-in-zoos-and-aquariums-damages-their-brains-142240
23. PETA. (2020). Animal Agriculture Increases the Risk of Pandemics. https://

References

www.peta.org/issues/animals-used-for-food/animals-used-food-factsheets/animal-agriculture-and-pandemics/

24. PETA. (2019). What Is Speciesism and How You Can Overcome It. https://www.peta.org/features/what-is-speciesism/
25. World Animal Protection. (2020). Animal Protection Index. https://api.worldanimalprotection.org/
26. Constitutional Rights Foundation. (2008). BRIA 24 1 b Upton Sinclair's The Jungle: Muckraking the Meat-Packing Industry. https://www.crf-usa.org/bill-of-rights-in-action/bria-24-1-b-upton-sinclairs-the-jungle-muckraking-the-meat-packing-industry.html
27. Moss, D.A. (2017). Democracy: A Case Study. https://www.jstor.org/stable/j.ctv31xf5x1
28. Human Rights Watch (Organization). (2004). Blood, Sweat, and Fear: Workers' Rights in U.S. Meat and Poultry Plants. https://www.fao.org/3/a0701e/a0701e.pdf
29. PETA Australia. (n.d.). Factory Farming Is a Human Rights Issue, Too. https://www.peta.org.au/issues/factory-farming-human-rights/
30. McSweeney, E. & Young, H. (2021). 'The Whole System Is Rotten': Life inside Europe's Meat Industry. https://www.theguardian.com/environment/2021/sep/28/the-whole-system-is-rotten-life-inside-europes-meat-industry
31. McSweeney, E. & Young, H. (2021). Revealed: Exploitation of Meat Plant Workers Rife across UK and Europe. https://www.theguardian.com/environment/2021/sep/28/revealed-exploitation-of-meat-plant-workers-rife-across-uk-and-europe
32. ETUC. (2021). Huge Fall in Labour Inspections Raises Covid Risk. https://www.etuc.org/en/pressrelease/huge-fall-labour-inspections-raises-covid-risk
33. ASPCA. (2018). New Investigation Highlights Dangers of High-Speed Slaughter. https://www.aspca.org/news/new-investigation-highlights-dangers-high-speed-slaughter
34. Scott-Reid, J. (2019). Advocates Agree: Increasing Kill Line Speeds Puts Animals and Workers at Risk. https://sentientmedia.org/advocates-agree-increasing-kill-line-speeds-puts-animals-and-workers-at-risk/
35. Richards, E., Signal, T., & Taylor, N. (2013). A Different Cut? Comparing Attitudes toward Animals and Propensity for Aggression within Two Primary Industry Cohorts—Farmers and Meatworkers. https://brill.com/view/journals/soan/21/4/article-p395_5.xml
36. PETA Australia. (2020). Does Australian Milk Contain Cow Poo? https://www.peta.org.au/news/milk-contains-poo/
37. ABC News. (2016). WA Milk Contamination Worries Spark Mass Recall. https://www.abc.net.au/news/2016-01-26/milk-recall-coles-wa-over-

microbial-contamination-fears/7115698
38. Greger, M. (2011). How Much Pus Is There in Milk? https://nutritionfacts.org/blog/how-much-pus-is-there-in-milk/
39. Consumer Reports. (2014). The High Cost of Cheap Chicken: 97 Percent of the Breasts We Tested Harbored Bacteria That Could Make You Sick. Learn How to Protect Yourself. https://www.dropbox.com/s/wfwjnj6u8i6hb8x/High%20Cost%20of%20Cheap%20Chicken.pdf?dl=0
40. PCRM. (2019). Doctors Sue USDA for Ignoring Concerns Over Fecal Contamination of Chicken. https://www.pcrm.org/news/news-releases/doctors-sue-usda-ignoring-concerns-over-fecal-contamination-chicken
41. Marchese, A. & Hovorka, A. (2022). Zoonoses Transfer, Factory Farms and Unsustainable Human–Animal Relations. https://www.mdpi.com/2071-1050/14/19/12806
42. Belk, A.D., Duarte, T., Quinn, C., et al. (2021). Air versus Water Chilling of Chicken: A Pilot Study of Quality, Shelf-Life, Microbial Ecology, and Economics. https://journals.asm.org/doi/10.1128/mSystems.00912-20
43. Loria, K. (2019). Poultry Processing Tech: The Art of Air Chilling. https://www.meatpoultry.com/articles/21769-poultry-processing-tech-the-art-of-air-chilling
44. Popham, P. (2000). How India's Sacred Cows Are Beaten, Abused and Poisoned to Make. https://www.independent.co.uk/news/world/asia/how-india-s-sacred-cows-are-beaten-abused-and-poisoned-to-make-leather-for-high-street-shops-724696.html
45. PETA. (2011). Animals in Entertainment: Circuses, SeaWorld, and Beyond. https://www.peta.org/issues/animals-in-entertainment/
46. Henn, C. (2020). The Shocking Truth About What Happens to 'Surplus' Zoo Animals. https://www.onegreenplanet.org/animalsandnature/the-shocking-truth-about-what-happens-to-surplus-zoo-animals/
47. Agence France-Presse. (2014). Danish Zoo That Killed Marius the Giraffe Puts down Four Lions. https://www.theguardian.com/world/2014/mar/25/danish-copenhagen-zoo-kills-four-lions-marius-giraffe
48. Schipani, S. (2019). The History of the Lab Rat Is Full of Scientific Triumphs and Ethical Quandaries. https://www.smithsonianmag.com/science-nature/history-lab-rat-scientific-triumphs-ethical-quandaries-180971533/
49. McAndrew, R. & Helms Tillery, S.I. (2016). Laboratory Primates: Their Lives in and after Research. https://www.ncbi.nlm.nih.gov/pmc/articles/PMC5198805/
50. Boyd, R. (2014). The Indigenous and Modern Relationship between People and Animals. https://www.resilience.org/stories/2014-01-17/the-indigenous-and-modern-relationship-between-people-and-animals/
51. Asia for Educators. (n.d.). Mongols in World History | The Pastoral

References

Nomadic Life. http://afe.easia.columbia.edu/mongols/pastoral/pastoral.htm
52. Bird, R.B., Tayor, N., Codding, B.F., et al. (2013). Niche Construction and Dreaming Logic: Aboriginal Patch Mosaic Burning and Varanid Lizards (Varanus Gouldii) in Australia. https://royalsocietypublishing.org/doi/10.1098/rspb.2013.2297
53. Dengler, R. (2019). Ancient Sri Lankans Figured Out How to Sustainably Hunt Monkeys and Squirrels. https://www.discovermagazine.com/planet-earth/ancient-sri-lankans-figured-out-how-to-sustainably-hunt-monkeys-and-squirrels
54. Our World in Data. (2021). Yearly Number of Animals Slaughtered for Meat, World, 1961 to 2021 (FAO). https://ourworldindata.org/meat-production#number-of-animals-slaughtered

Chapter 3

1. Fowler, J.H. & Christakis, N.A. (2008). Dynamic Spread of Happiness in a Large Social Network: Longitudinal Analysis over 20 Years in the Framingham Heart Study. https://www.bmj.com/lookup/doi/10.1136/bmj.a2338
2. Mednick, S.C., Christakis, N.A., & Fowler, J.H. (2010). The Spread of Sleep Loss Influences Drug Use in Adolescent Social Networks. https://journals.plos.org/plosone/article?id=10.1371/journal.pone.0009775
3. Rosenquist, J.N., Fowler, J.H., & Christakis, N.A. (2011). Social Network Determinants of Depression. https://www.nature.com/articles/mp201013
4. Expert Participants. (1947). Agriculture Act 1947-10 & 11 Geo. 6, Chap, 48. https://www.legislation.gov.uk/ukpga/Geo6/10-11/48
5. European Commission. (2023). The Common Agricultural Policy at a Glance. https://agriculture.ec.europa.eu/common-agricultural-policy/cap-overview/cap-glance_en
6. Evans, M. (2017). Do We Eat Too Much Meat? https://www.sbs.com.au/food/article/do-we-eat-too-much-meat/lebccl2zf
7. Our World in Data. (2021). Yearly Number of Animals Slaughtered for Meat, World, 1961 to 2021 (FAO). https://ourworldindata.org/meat-production#number-of-animals-slaughtered
8. Joyce, C. (2010). Food For Thought: Meat-Based Diet Made Us Smarter. https://www.npr.org/2010/08/02/128849908/food-for-thought-meat-based-diet-made-us-smarter
9. The University of Sydney. (2015). Starchy Carbs, Not a Paleo Diet, Advanced the Human Race. https://www.sydney.edu.au/news-opinion/news/2015/08/10/starchy-carbs--not-a-paleo-diet--advanced-the-human-race.html
10. University Of Minnesota. (1999). Light My Fire: Cooking As Key

To Modern Human Evolution. https://www.sciencedaily.com/releases/1999/08/990810064914.htm
11. Pennisi, E. (1999). Did Cooked Tubers Spur the Evolution of Big Brains? https://www.science.org/doi/10.1126/science.283.5410.2004
12. Mariotti, F. & Gardner, C.D. (2019). Dietary Protein and Amino Acids in Vegetarian Diets—A Review. https://www.ncbi.nlm.nih.gov/pmc/articles/PMC6893534/
13. Gardner, C., Hartle, J., Garrett, R., et al. (2019). Maximizing the Intersection of Human Health and the Health of the Environment with Regard to the Amount and Type of Protein Produced and Consumed in the United States. https://www.researchgate.net/publication/331560091_Maximizing_the_intersection_of_human_health_and_the_health_of_the_environment_with_regard_to_the_amount_and_type_of_protein_produced_and_consumed_in_the_United_States
14. Piedmont Healthcare. (n.d.). What Is a Complete Protein? https://www.piedmont.org/living-better/what-is-a-complete-protein
15. Rose, M. (2021). Soy-Chosis: The Strange but True Origin of How a Bean Became Demonized by a Nation (and Beyond). https://marla-rose.medium.com/soy-chosis-the-strange-but-true-origin-of-how-a-bean-became-demonized-by-a-nation-and-beyond-22b1f124ac11
16. Setchell, K.D., Brown, N.M., Zhao, X., et al. (2011). Soy Isoflavone Phase II Metabolism Differs between Rodents and Humans: Implications for the Effect on Breast Cancer Risk. https://www.ncbi.nlm.nih.gov/pmc/articles/PMC3192476/
17. ASCO Staff. (2021). Can Eating Soy Cause Breast Cancer? https://www.cancer.net/blog/2021-10/can-eating-soy-cause-breast-cancer
18. Patisaul, H.B. & Jefferson, W. (2010). The Pros and Cons of Phytoestrogens. https://www.ncbi.nlm.nih.gov/pmc/articles/PMC3074428/
19. Reed, K.E., Camargo, J., Hamilton-Reeves, J., et al. (2021). Neither Soy nor Isoflavone Intake Affects Male Reproductive Hormones: An Expanded and Updated Meta-Analysis of Clinical Studies. https://pubmed.ncbi.nlm.nih.gov/33383165/
20. Willett, W. (2022). Ask a Doctor: Is Animal Protein Easier to Absorb than Plant Protein? https://www.washingtonpost.com/wellness/2022/10/31/animal-plant-protein-absorption-digestion/
21. SCIMEX. (2015). Red Meat Linked to Cancer – WHO Report. https://www.scimex.org/newsfeed/red-meat-and-cancer-iarc-report
22. Cancer Council NSW. (n.d.). Red Meat, Processed Meat and Cancer. https://www.cancercouncil.com.au/1in3cancers/lifestyle-choices-and-cancer/red-meat-processed-meat-and-cancer/
23. Song, M., Fung, T.T., Hu, F.B., et al. (2016). Association of Animal and

References

Plant Protein Intake With All-Cause and Cause-Specific Mortality. https://pubmed.ncbi.nlm.nih.gov/27479196/

24. Huang, J., Liao, L.M., Weinstein, S.J., et al. (2020). Association Between Plant and Animal Protein Intake and Overall and Cause-Specific Mortality. https://doi.org/10.1001/jamainternmed.2020.2790
25. McHutchison, T. (2014). Paleo Says No to Grains. But Is It Justified? https://blogs.deakin.edu.au/deakinnutrition/2014/02/26/paleo-says-no-to-grains-but-is-it-justified/
26. Harvard T.H. Chan School of Public Health. (2019). Are Anti-Nutrients Harmful? https://www.hsph.harvard.edu/nutritionsource/anti-nutrients/
27. Curhan, G.C., Willett, W.C., Knight, E.L., et al. (2004). Dietary Factors and the Risk of Incident Kidney Stones in Younger Women: Nurses' Health Study II. https://pubmed.ncbi.nlm.nih.gov/15111375/
28. Burckhardt, P. (2015). Calcium Revisited, Part III: Effect of Dietary Calcium on BMD and Fracture Risk. https://pubmed.ncbi.nlm.nih.gov/26331006/
29. Feskanich, D., Willett, W.C., Stampfer, M.J., et al. (1997). Milk, Dietary Calcium, and Bone Fractures in Women: A 12-Year Prospective Study. https://pubmed.ncbi.nlm.nih.gov/9224182/
30. Feskanich, D., Bischoff-Ferrari, H.A., Frazier, A.L., et al. (2014). Milk Consumption during Teenage Years and Risk of Hip Fractures in Older Adults. https://pubmed.ncbi.nlm.nih.gov/24247817/
31. Sonneville, K.R., Gordon, C.M., Kocher, M.S., et al. (2012). Vitamin D, Calcium, and Dairy Intakes and Stress Fractures Among Female Adolescents. https://jamanetwork.com/journals/jamapediatrics/fullarticle/1149502
32. Chan, J.M., Stampfer, M.J., Ma, J., et al. (2001). Dairy Products, Calcium, and Prostate Cancer Risk in the Physicians' Health Study. https://pubmed.ncbi.nlm.nih.gov/11566656/
33. Kurlansky, M. (2018). Milk!: A 10,000-Year Food Fracas. https://www.amazon.com.au/Milk-10-000-Year-Food-Fracas/dp/1632863820
34. Hamilton, A. (2016). Got Milked?: The Great Dairy Deception and Why You'll Thrive Without Milk. https://www.amazon.com.au/Got-Milked-Deception-Thrive-Without/dp/0062362089
35. Stukenberg, D., Blayney, D., & Miller, J. (2006). Major Advances in Milk Marketing: Government and Industry Consolidation. https://www.sciencedirect.com/science/article/pii/S0022030206721890
36. Rainey, C. (2017). These Cheese Scientists Are Fighting to Save the Dairy Industry. https://www.bloomberg.com/news/features/2017-07-19/the-mad-cheese-scientists-fighting-to-save-the-dairy-industry
37. O'Connell, J. (1990). 1990 Milk, Calcium and Osteoporosis. https://australianfoodtimeline.com.au/osteoporosis/
38. Media Watch. (2023). Dairy Spin. https://www.facebook.com/

watch/?v=1346293926235166
39. Smith, M., Love, D.C., Rochman, C.M., et al. (2018). Microplastics in Seafood and the Implications for Human Health. https://www.ncbi.nlm.nih.gov/pmc/articles/PMC6132564/
40. Barboza, L.G.A., Lopes, C., Oliveira, P., et al. (2020). Microplastics in Wild Fish from North East Atlantic Ocean and Its Potential for Causing Neurotoxic Effects, Lipid Oxidative Damage, and Human Health Risks Associated with Ingestion Exposure. https://www.sciencedirect.com/science/article/pii/S0048969719346169
41. Guilford, G. (2015). Here's Why Your Farmed Salmon Has Color Added to It. https://qz.com/358811/heres-why-your-farmed-salmon-has-color-added-to-it
42. Brockway, O. & Brockway, L. (2022). Eating Our Way To Extinction | The Documentary. https://www.eating2extinction.com/
43. Tabrizi, A. (2021). Seaspiracy Facts. https://www.seaspiracy.org/facts
44. Rise of The Vegan. (2017). B12: Why It's Not Just a Vegan Issue. https://www.riseofthevegan.com/blog/b12-is-not-just-a-vegan-problem
45. Mayo Clinic Staff. (n.d.). Vitamin B-12. https://www.mayoclinic.org/drugs-supplements-vitamin-b12/art-20363663
46. Harvard T.H. Chan School of Public Health. (2019). Iron. https://www.hsph.harvard.edu/nutritionsource/iron/
47. Zielinski, L. (2019). Selenium Benefits: Here Are 7 That Are Proven by Science. https://ro.co/health-guide/selenium-benefits/
48. Eske, J. (2019). Brazil Nuts: Health Benefits, Nutrition, and Risks. https://www.medicalnewstoday.com/articles/325000
49. Cleveland Clinic. (2022). Iodine Deficiency: Symptoms, Causes, Treatment & Prevention. https://my.clevelandclinic.org/health/diseases/23417-iodine-deficiency
50. Saunders, A.V., Craig, W.J., & Baines, S.K. (2013). Zinc and Vegetarian Diets. https://www.mja.com.au/journal/2013/199/4/zinc-and-vegetarian-diets
51. Dickens, R. (2020). Zinc Rich Foods For Vegetarians. https://racheldickens.ca/general-nutrition/zinc-rich-foods-for-vegetarians/
52. PNW & D'Andrea, G. (2020). Vegan Zinc Sources, Absorption, and Deficiency | PNW. https://www.plantnutritionwellness.com/vegan-zinc-sources-absorption-and-deficiency/
53. Kaviani, M., Shaw, K., & Chilibeck, P.D. (2020). Benefits of Creatine Supplementation for Vegetarians Compared to Omnivorous Athletes: A Systematic Review. https://www.ncbi.nlm.nih.gov/pmc/articles/PMC7246861/
54. Hill, S. (2021). The Proof Is in the Plants: How Science Shows a Plant-

References

Based Diet Could Save Your Life. https://www.amazon.com.au/Proof-Plants-science-plant-based-planet-ebook/dp/B085ZZ21RG
55. Hill, S. (2023). Fact-Check #4: Paul Saladino on Grains and Legumes. https://www.youtube.com/watch?v=iNy1whdSgtA
56. Key, T.J., Papier, K., & Tong, T.Y.N. (2022). Plant-Based Diets and Long-Term Health: Findings from the EPIC-Oxford Study. https://pubmed.ncbi.nlm.nih.gov/35934687/
57. Oxford Population Health. (n.d.). EPIC-Oxford. https://www.ceu.ox.ac.uk/research/epic-oxford-1/epic-oxford
58. Buettner, D. & Skemp, S. (2016). Blue Zones. https://www.ncbi.nlm.nih.gov/pmc/articles/PMC6125071/
59. Willett, W., Rockström, J., Loken, B., et al. (2019). Food in the Anthropocene: The EAT–Lancet Commission on Healthy Diets from Sustainable Food Systems. https://www.thelancet.com/journals/lancet/article/PIIS0140-6736(18)31788-4/fulltext
60. EAT. (n.d.). EAT-Lancet Commission on Food, Planet, Health. https://eatforum.org/eat-lancet-commission/
61. McCormick, B. (2019). What do the Biggest Nutrition Organisations Say About Veganism? https://vomad.life/nutrients/
62. Clarke, C. (2020). David Attenborough: A Life on Our Planet Review – Stark Climate Emergency Warning. http://www.theguardian.com/film/2020/sep/25/david-attenborough-a-life-on-our-planet-review-climate-emergency-documentary
63. McNulty, R. (2019). Arnold Schwarzenegger Advocates for Plant-Based Diets in New Documentary. https://www.muscleandfitness.com/athletes-celebrities/news/arnold-schwarzenegger-advocates-plant-based-diets-new-documentary/
64. PopulationU. (2023). Countries by GDP 2023. https://www.populationu.com/gen/countries-by-gdp
65. Shahbandeh, M. (2022). Global Meat Industry - Statistics & Facts. https://www.statista.com/topics/4880/global-meat-industry/
66. Crowley, J., Ball, L., & Hiddink, G.J. (2019). Nutrition in Medical Education: A Systematic Review. https://www.thelancet.com/journals/lanplh/article/PIIS2542-51961930171-8/fulltext
67. Factory Farming Awareness & O'Keefe, J. (2022). How the Meat and Dairy Industry Fund Scientific Research. https://ffacoalition.org/articles/meat-money-how-the-meat-and-dairy-industry-fund-scientific-research/
68. Almendral, A. (2023). The Meat Industry Blocked the IPCC's Attempt to Recommend a Plant-Based Diet. https://qz.com/ipcc-report-on-climate-change-meat-industry-1850261179
69. USDA ERS. (2023). Dairy: Policy. https://www.ers.usda.gov/topics/animal-

products/dairy/policy/
70. Duhaime-Ross, A. (2016). New US Food Guidelines Show the Power of Lobbying, Not Science. https://www.theverge.com/2016/1/7/10726606/2015-us-dietary-guidelines-meat-and-soda-lobbying-power
71. Moran, G. (2021). Questions Remain about Big Food's Influence on the New Dietary Guidelines. https://civileats.com/2021/01/28/questions-remain-about-big-foods-influence-on-the-new-dietary-guidelines/
72. DeSmog. (n.d.). Agriculture and Horticulture Development Board. https://www.desmog.com/agriculture-horticulture-development-board/
73. British Nutrition Foundation. (n.d.). Who We Work With. https://www.nutrition.org.uk/our-work/who-we-work-with/
74. Simon, M. (2015). Is the Dietitians Association of Australia in the Pocket of Big Food? https://www.eatdrinkpolitics.com/wp-content/uploads/DAAReportEatDrinkPolitics.pdf
75. Health Canada. (2019). Canada's Dietary Guidelines. https://food-guide.canada.ca/sites/default/files/artifact-pdf/CDG-EN-2018.pdf
76. Joy, M. (2011). Why We Love Dogs, Eat Pigs, and Wear Cows: An Introduction to Carnism. https://www.amazon.com/Love-Dogs-Pigs-Wear-Cows/dp/1573245054
77. Dixon, F. (2022). Are Humans Herbivores or Omnivores? https://nutritionstudies.org/are-humans-herbivores-or-omnivores/
78. Cowell, A. (1992). After 350 Years, Vatican Says Galileo Was Right: It Moves. https://www.nytimes.com/1992/10/31/world/after-350-years-vatican-says-galileo-was-right-it-moves.html
79. Davis, R. (2015). The Doctor Who Championed Hand-Washing and Briefly Saved Lives. https://www.npr.org/sections/health-shots/2015/01/12/375663920/the-doctor-who-championed-hand-washing-and-saved-women-s-lives
80. Olvera, L. (2020). Marketing Masculinity: The Meat of the Matter. https://sentientmedia.org/marketing-masculinity-the-meat-of-the-matter/
81. Pohlmann, A. (2014). Threatened at the Table: Meat Consumption, Maleness and Men's Gender Identities. http://hdl.handle.net/10125/100470
82. Hillier, D. (2022). Meet the 'Vegan Bros' Here to Bust the Myth That Real Men Eat Meat. https://www.theguardian.com/lifeandstyle/2022/mar/05/vegan-bros-busting-myth-that-real-men-eat-meat
83. Owyoung, P. (2022). Men, Meat, and the Marketing of Manhood. https://goodmenproject.com/featured-content/men-meat-and-the-marketing-of-manhood/
84. Bray, H.J., Zambrano, S.C., Chur-Hansen, A., et al. (2016). Not Appropriate Dinner Table Conversation? Talking to Children about Meat Production. https://pubmed.ncbi.nlm.nih.gov/26806026/

References

85. Ascione, F.R. (1993). Children Who Are Cruel to Animals: A Review of Research and Implications for Developmental Psychopathology. https://doi.org/10.2752/089279393787002105
86. Smithers, R. (2017). Tesco Faces Legal Threat over Marketing Its Food with "Fake Farm" Names. https://www.theguardian.com/environment/2017/dec/13/tesco-faces-legal-threat-over-marketing-its-food-with-fake-farm-names
87. Reese, J. (2018). There's No Such Thing as Humane Meat or Eggs. Stop Kidding Yourself. https://www.theguardian.com/food/2018/nov/16/theres-no-such-thing-as-humane-meat-or-eggs-stop-kidding-yourself
88. McGreal, C. (2019). How America's Food Giants Swallowed the Family Farms. https://www.theguardian.com/environment/2019/mar/09/american-food-giants-swallow-the-family-farms-iowa
89. Peterson Farm Brothers. (n.d.). Are There Still Family Farmers? Or Are Most Farms Factory Farms and Industrial Farms? https://petersonfarmbrothers.com/are-there-still-family-farmers-or-are-most-farms-factory-farms-and-industrial-farms/
90. Thomas Foods Feedlot. (2022). Thomas Foods Feedlot. https://www.facebook.com/tfi.feedlot/posts/pfbid0NaxExhgR2hZSruxF3ckndeQbjTPzm3tPSgdWJaaxLXA1GbGiFxwateERijvuY49dl
91. TFI. (2023). About TFI. https://thomasfoods.com/about-us/
92. Berry, K. (2020). Thomas Foods Expands and Rebrands. https://www.foodanddrinkbusiness.com.au/news/thomas-foods-expands-and-rebrands
93. ACMF. (n.d.). Free Range, RSPCA, Organic – What Are the Differences? https://www.chicken.org.au/chicken-meat-production/
94. CHOICE staff. (2021). Are Your Eggs Really Free-Range? https://www.choice.com.au/food-and-drink/meat-fish-and-eggs/eggs/articles/what-free-range-eggs-meet-the-model-code
95. CHOICE staff. (2019). Meat Reviews, Tests, Information and Buying Guides. https://www.choice.com.au/food-and-drink/meat-fish-and-eggs/meat
96. Purewal, A.K. (2022). New Zealand Farming Production Systems – Pigs. https://ahdb.org.uk/trade-and-policy-New-Zealand-farming-production-systems-pigs
97. Pasture for Life. (n.d.). Pasture for Life – FAQs. https://www.pastureforlife.org/faqs/
98. Sustainable Table. (2023). Let's Talk Beef. https://www.sustainabletable.org.au/journal/beef
99. Rivera, L. (2017). The Truth Behind the Pork We Eat. https://www.independent.co.uk/life-style/food-and-drink/pork-production-truth-pig-farming-uk-factory-hughfearnley-whittingstall-sienna-miller-mick-jagger-a7813746.html

100. Winters, E. (2022). This Is Vegan Propaganda: (& Other Lies the Meat Industry Tells You). https://www.amazon.com.au/This-Vegan-Propaganda-Other-Industry/dp/1785043765
101. Sanders, B. (2020). Global Animal Slaughter Statistics & Charts: 2020 Update. https://faunalytics.org/global-animal-slaughter-statistics-and-charts-2020-update/
102. Meat & Livestock Australia. (2021). Grainfed Cattle Make up 50% of Beef Production. https://www.mla.com.au/prices-markets/market-news/2021/grainfed-cattle-make-up-50-of-beef-production/
103. Australian Pork. (n.d.). Indoor System Farming. https://australianpork.com.au/about-pig-farming/indoor-system-farming
104. PETA Australia. (n.d.). The Truth About Chickens Used for Meat in Australia - Issues. https://www.peta.org.au/issues/food/truth-chickens-food/
105. Cervera, M. (2022). Investigation Reveals UK Has over 1,000 Mega-Farms in Livestock-Intensive Farming Boom. https://www.foodingredientsfirst.com/news/investigation-reveals-uk-has-over-1000-mega-farms-in-livestock-intensive-farming-boom.html
106. Wasley, A. & Kroeker, H. (2018). Revealed: Industrial-Scale Beef Farming Comes to the UK. https://www.theguardian.com/environment/2018/may/29/revealed-industrial-scale-beef-farming-comes-to-the-uk
107. Shelling, M. (2018). Clean Green Beef No Longer on Our Menu? How Feedlots Are Changing the Face of the New Zealand Agri-Food System. https://www.thebigq.org/2018/10/30/clean-green-beef-no-longer-on-our-menu-how-feedlots-are-changing-the-face-of-the-new-zealand-agri-food-system/
108. Mathus, N. (2018). M. Bovis Hits Beef Feedlot. https://www.ruralnewsgroup.co.nz/rural-news/rural-general-news/m-bovis-hits-beef-feedlot
109. Eating Better. (2020). We Need to Talk about Chicken. https://www.eating-better.org/uploads/Documents/2020/EB_WeNeedToTalkAboutChicken_Feb20_A4_Final.pdf
110. RSPCA. (n.d.). Pig Farming in the UK. http://www.rspca.org.uk/adviceandwelfare/farm/pigs/farming
111. Safe. (n.d.). Free Range. https://safe.org.nz/our-work/animals-in-aotearoa/intensive-farming__trashed/free-range/
112. Reddy, J. (2022). Pig Farming in New Zealand: Breeds, How to Start. https://www.agrifarming.in/pig-farming-in-new-zealand-breeds-how-to-start
113. Harvey, F. (2021). Fewer, Bigger, More Intensive: EU Vows to Stem Drastic Loss of Small Farms. https://www.theguardian.com/environment/2021/

References

may/24/fewer-bigger-more-intensive-eu-vows-to-stem-drastic-loss-of-small-farms

114. The Science Agriculture. (n.d.). Livestock Archives. https://scienceagri.com/category/livestock/
115. Bechtel, W. (2018). Cattle on Feed Numbers: A Look Around the World. https://www.drovers.com/markets/cattle-feed-numbers-look-around-world
116. Animal Clock. (2023). 2023 U.S. Animal Kill Clock. http://animalclock.org
117. Delforce, C. (2018). Dominion. https://www.imdb.com/title/tt5773402/
118. Winters, E. & Woods, L. (2017). Land of Hope and Glory. https://www.imdb.com/title/tt7214598/
119. Anthis, J.R. (2019). US Factory Farming Estimates. https://sentienceinstitute.org/us-factory-farming-estimates
120. Kirby, M. (2013). Factory Farming Masks Meat's True Costs. https://www.abc.net.au/news/2013-06-21/kirby-modern-meat/4770226
121. Corselo. (2018). Archive: Small and Large Farms in the EU - Statistics from the Farm Structure Survey. https://ec.europa.eu/eurostat/statistics-explained/index.php?title=Archive:Small_and_large_farms_in_the_EU_-_statistics_from_the_farm_structure_survey
122. Farm Transparency Project. (2019). Farm Transparency Map: Interactive Map of Australian Factory Farms and Slaughterhouses. https://www.farmtransparency.org/map
123. CounterGlow. (n.d.). CounterGlow Map. https://map.counterglow.org/
124. Poultry Hub Australia. (n.d.). Meat Chicken (Broiler) Industry. https://www.poultryhub.org/production/meat-chicken-broiler-industry
125. Voiceless. (n.d.). Ag-Gag Laws in Australia. https://voiceless.org.au/hot-topics/ag-gag/
126. Batheja, A. (2018). The Time Oprah Winfrey Beefed with the Texas Cattle Industry. https://www.texastribune.org/2018/01/10/time-oprah-winfrey-beefed-texas-cattle-industry/
127. Etymonline. (2019). Meat. https://www.etymonline.com/word/meat
128. Clarke, J. (2017). In the Middle Ages, the Upper Class Went Nuts for Almond Milk. http://www.atlasobscura.com/articles/almond-milk-obsession-origins-middle-ages
129. FRSC. (2019). Misleading Descriptions for Food Options Paper. https://www.health.gov.au/sites/default/files/documents/2020/04/foi-request-1456-food-labelling-misleading-descriptions-for-food-options-paper.pdf
130. Gleckel, J.A. (2020). Are Consumers Really Confused by Plant-Based Food Labels? An Empirical Study. https://papers.ssrn.com/abstract=3727710

131. Whipple, T. (2023). Meat Farmers Likened to Big Tobacco for Downplaying Risks to Health. https://www.thetimes.co.uk/article/meat-farmers-likened-to-big-tobacco-for-downplaying-risks-to-health-0n288rfs7
132. Stanescu, V. (2019). "Cowgate": Meat Eating and Climate Change Denial. *Climate Change Denial and Public Relations*. https://www.taylorfrancis.com/chapters/oa-edit/10.4324/9781351121798-11/cowgate-vasile-stanescu
133. OpenSecrets. (2023). Sector Profile: Agribusiness. https://www.opensecrets.org/federal-lobbying/sectors/summary?id=A
134. Lazarus, O., McDermid, S., & Jacquet, J. (2021). The Climate Responsibilities of Industrial Meat and Dairy Producers. https://link.springer.com/10.1007/s10584-021-03047-7
135. CEAP. (2021). Research Brief #5: The Climate Responsibilities of Industrial Meat and Dairy Producers. https://s18798.pcdn.co/ceap/wp-content/uploads/sites/11111/2021/04/CEAP_Research_Brief_5.pdf
136. Dunne, D. (2021). Global Meat Industry 'Using Tobacco Company Tactics' to Downplay Role in Driving Climate Crisis, Investigation Claims. https://www.independent.co.uk/climate-change/news/meat-dairy-industry-greenwashing-climate-b1884769.html
137. McKie, R.E. (2019). Climate Change Counter Movement Neutralization Techniques: A Typology to Examine the Climate Change Counter Movement. https://onlinelibrary.wiley.com/doi/10.1111/soin.12246
138. Ritchie, H. (2020). You Want to Reduce the Carbon Footprint of Your Food? Focus on What You Eat, Not Whether Your Food Is Local. https://ourworldindata.org/food-choice-vs-eating-local
139. Scarborough, P., Appleby, P.N., Mizdrak, A., et al. (2014). Dietary Greenhouse Gas Emissions of Meat-Eaters, Fish-Eaters, Vegetarians and Vegans in the UK. https://doi.org/10.1007/s10584-014-1169-1
140. Weber, C.L. & Matthews, H.S. (2008). Food-Miles and the Relative Climate Impacts of Food Choices in the United States. https://doi.org/10.1021/es702969f
141. Pieper, M., Michalke, A., & Gaugler, T. (2020). Calculation of External Climate Costs for Food Highlights Inadequate Pricing of Animal Products. https://www.nature.com/articles/s41467-020-19474-6
142. Smith, L.G., Kirk, G.J.D., Jones, P.J., et al. (2019). The Greenhouse Gas Impacts of Converting Food Production in England and Wales to Organic Methods. https://www.nature.com/articles/s41467-019-12622-7
143. FAO. (2018). The State of World Fisheries and Aquaculture 2018: Meeting the Sustainable Development Goals. https://www.fao.org/3/i9540en/I9540EN.pdf

References

144. Myers, R.A. & Worm, B. (2003). Rapid Worldwide Depletion of Predatory Fish Communities. https://www.nature.com/articles/nature01610
145. MSC. (n.d.). Sustainable Fishing | MSC. https://www.msc.org
146. Willow, F. (2019). Is MSC Certified Fish Really Sustainable? https://ethicalunicorn.com/2019/02/22/is-msc-certified-fish-really-sustainable/
147. Openseas. (2018). Scallop Dredging: Eco-Label the Problems Away. https://www.openseas.org.uk/news/scallop-dredging-eco-label-the-problems-away/
148. McVeigh, K. (2021). Blue Ticked off: The Controversy over the MSC Fish 'Ecolabel.' https://www.theguardian.com/environment/2021/jul/26/blue-ticked-off-the-controversy-over-the-msc-fish-ecolabel
149. Marine Conservation Society. (2023). How Our Good Fish Guide Ratings Work. https://www.mcsuk.org/ocean-emergency/sustainable-seafood/the-good-fish-guide/how-our-good-fish-guide-ratings-work/
150. Miller, M. (2020). Farm Babe: USDA's "Grass Fed" Beef Label may not be What it Seems. https://www.agdaily.com/livestock/farm-babe-usdas-grass-fed-beef-label-may-not-be-what-it-seems/
151. Ranganathan, J., Waite, R., Searchinger, T., et al. (2020). Regenerative Agriculture: Good for Soil Health, but Limited Potential to Mitigate Climate Change. https://www.wri.org/insights/regenerative-agriculture-good-soil-health-limited-potential-mitigate-climate-change
152. Lewis, T. (2021). 'Sustainable Isn't a Thing': Why Regenerative Agriculture Is Food's Latest Buzzword. https://www.theguardian.com/food/2021/jul/18/sustainable-isnt-a-thing-why-regenerative-agriculture-is-foods-latest-buzzword
153. Garnett, T. (2017). Why Eating Grass-Fed Beef Isn't Going to Help Fight Climate Change. http://theconversation.com/why-eating-grass-fed-beef-isnt-going-to-help-fight-climate-change-84237
154. Garnett, T., Godde, C., Muller, A., et al. (2017). Grazed and Confused?: Ruminating on Cattle, Grazing Systems, Methane, Nitrous Oxide, the Soil Carbon Sequestration Question-and What It All Means for Greenhouse Gas Emissions. https://www.tabledebates.org/sites/default/files/2020-10/fcrn_gnc_report.pdf
155. Smith, P. (2014). Do Grasslands Act as a Perpetual Sink for Carbon? https://onlinelibrary.wiley.com/doi/abs/10.1111/gcb.12561
156. Norman, C. & Kreye, M. (2020). How Forests Store Carbon. https://extension.psu.edu/how-forests-store-carbon
157. Campbell, L. (2019). Grass-Fed Beef: Is It Really a Sustainable Alternative? https://nutritionstudies.org/grass-fed-beef-a-sustainable-alternative/

158. Hayek, M.N. & Garrett, R.D. (2018). Nationwide Shift to Grass-Fed Beef Requires Larger Cattle Population. https://iopscience.iop.org/article/10.1088/1748-9326/aad401
159. Hill, S.J. (2021). Can Holistic Grazing Reverse Climate Change? https://theproof.com/can-holistic-grazing-reverse-climate-change/
160. Ritchie, H., Rodés-Guirao, L., Mathieu, E., et al. (2023). Population Growth. https://ourworldindata.org/population-growth
161. WWF. (2018). What Are the Biggest Drivers of Tropical Deforestation? https://www.worldwildlife.org/magazine/issues/summer-2018/articles/what-are-the-biggest-drivers-of-tropical-deforestation

Chapter 4

1. Foer, J.S. (2019). We Are the Weather: Saving the Planet Begins at Breakfast. https://www.amazon.com.au/We-Are-Weather-Saving-Breakfast/dp/0374280002
2. Porter, M. (2022). 7 Scary Ingredients Hiding in Your Halloween Treats - Animal Save Movement. https://thesavemovement.org/7-scary-ingredients-hiding-in-your-halloween-treats/
3. The Kind Store. (2023). 15 Non-Vegan Ingredients to Avoid in Your Skincare. https://www.thekindstoreonline.co.uk/blogs/blog/non-vegan-ingredients-to-avoid-in-skincare
4. Güler Tuck, Z. (2021). 20 Surprising Things That Contain Animal Products. https://medium.com/the-b/20-surprising-things-that-contain-animal-products-69dd709fc1bc
5. Petroff, A. (2016). It's Not Just the U.K. These Countries Also Have Animal Fat in Their Money. https://money.cnn.com/2016/11/30/news/animal-fat-money-notes-bills-cash-australia-canada/index.html
6. Meixner, M. (2020). Is Alcohol Vegan? A Complete Guide to Beer, Wine, and Spirits. https://www.healthline.com/nutrition/is-alcohol-vegan
7. Barnivore. (n.d.). Is Your Booze Vegan? https://www.barnivore.com/
8. Jayathilakan, K., Sultana, K., Radhakrishna, K., et al. (2012). Utilization of Byproducts and Waste Materials from Meat, Poultry and Fish Processing Industries: A Review. https://www.ncbi.nlm.nih.gov/pmc/articles/PMC3614052/
9. Henchion, M., McCarthy, M., & O'Callaghan, J. (2016). Transforming Beef By-Products into Valuable Ingredients: Which Spell/Recipe to Use? https://www.frontiersin.org/articles/10.3389/fnut.2016.00053
10. Alao, B.O., Falowo, A.B., Chulayo, A., et al. (2017). The Potential of Animal By-Products in Food Systems: Production, Prospects and Challenges. https://www.mdpi.com/2071-1050/9/7/1089
11. Rogers, K. (2020). Want to Eat Less Meat? Take a Page from These

References

Cultures That Already Do. https://www.cnn.com/travel/article/vegetarian-diet-beginners-coronavirus-wellness/index.html

Chapter 5
1. Netherworld. (n.d.). Diner Bites + Buns + Bowls + Desserts. https://www.netherworldarcade.com/food/
2. Tzeses, J. (2020). Cognitive Dissonance: What It Is & Why It Matters. https://www.psycom.net/cognitive-dissonance
3. Murphy, L. (2015). How Social Proof Actually Works in Marketing. https://sixteenventures.com/social-proof
4. Mcleod, S. (2022). What Is Conformity? Definition, Types, Psychology Research. https://www.simplypsychology.org/conformity.html
5. Asch, S.E. (1956). Studies of Independence and Conformity: I. a Minority of One Against a Unanimous Majority. https://psycnet.apa.org/doiLanding?doi=10.1037/h0093718
6. Kahneman, D. (2013). Thinking, Fast and Slow. https://www.amazon.com.au/Thinking-Fast-Slow-Daniel-Kahneman/dp/0374533555
7. Shatz, I. (2016). The Confirmation Bias: Why People See What They Want to See. https://effectiviology.com/confirmation-bias/
8. Hassan, A. & Barber, S.J. (2021). The Effects of Repetition Frequency on the Illusory Truth Effect. https://doi.org/10.1186/s41235-021-00301-5
9. BehavioralEconomics. (2023). Sunk Cost Fallacy. https://www.behavioraleconomics.com/resources/mini-encyclopedia-of-be/sunk-cost-fallacy/
10. Fulkerson, L. (2013). Forks Over Knives. https://www.forksoverknives.com/the-film/
11. Farm Transitions Australia. (n.d.). Farm Transitions Australia. https://www.farmtransitionsaustralia.org/
12. RAP. (2022). Home. https://rancheradvocacy.org/
13. Sutton, J. (2016). What Is Willpower? The Psychology Behind Self-Control. https://positivepsychology.com/psychology-of-willpower/
14. Schaffner, A.K. (2020). Living With the Inner Critic: 8 Helpful Worksheets. https://positivepsychology.com/inner-critic-worksheets/

Chapter 6
1. Wright, N. (2018). Jordan Missed 9,000 Times. https://medium.com/striving-strategically/jordan-missed-9-000-times-ced3bea79c66
2. Ivereigh, A. (2016). Mother Teresa and the Media: What the Camera Saw. https://cruxnow.com/canonization-of-mother-teresa/2016/09/mother-teresa-media-camera-saw/
3. Coelho do Vale, R., Pieters, R., & Zeelenberg, M. (2016). The Benefits

of Behaving Badly on Occasion: Successful Regulation by Planned Hedonic Deviations. https://onlinelibrary.wiley.com/doi/abs/10.1016/j.jcps.2015.05.001
4. The Vegan Society. (n.d.). Definition of Veganism. https://www.vegansociety.com/go-vegan/definition-veganism
5. Impossible Foods. (2018). Setting the Record Straight: How PETA Extremists Are Undermining Their Own Mission. https://assets.ctfassets.net/hhv516v5f7sj/q95roYbzJAMea22kkiwQ2/7256a4ab2c24d0ea4a903991ba7150b1/PETA_The_Unofficial_Correction_FINAL.pdf
6. Chiorando, M. (2017). Impossible Foods CEO Speaks Out Over Animal Testing Row: "It Was An Agonizing Decision." https://plantbasednews.org/lifestyle/impossible-foods-ceo-blasts-animal-testing-i-abhor-the-exploitation-of-animals/
7. Sogari, G., Caputo, V., Joshua Petterson, A., et al. (2023). A Sensory Study on Consumer Valuation for Plant-Based Meat Alternatives: What Is Liked and Disliked the Most? https://www.sciencedirect.com/science/article/pii/S0963996923003587
8. Goodful. (2020). Impossible Burger Blind Taste Test. https://www.facebook.com/watch/?v=369461870873626
9. Slickdeals. (2021). "BLIND" TASTE TEST: Beyond, Impossible and Beef Burgers! https://www.youtube.com/watch?v=NYOCv-y8ckM
10. Khan, S., Loyola, C., Dettling, J., et al. (2019). Comparative Environmental LCA of the Impossible Burger with Conventional Ground Beef Burger. https://assets.ctfassets.net/hhv516v5f7sj/4exF7Ex74UoYku640WSF3t/cc213b148ee80fa2d8062e430012ec56/Impossible_foods_comparative_LCA.pdf
11. Impossible Foods. (2017). An Open Letter from Our CEO To Our Community. https://www.facebook.com/ImpossibleFoods/posts/pfbid074PQM1ZyGxUq3RxTGPiQmtiXprxRVbVWipYzMay5Ygqsu6YRCKui67pxwmA5TRRCl
12. Impossible Foods. (2017). The Agonizing Dilemma Of Animal Testing. https://webcache.googleusercontent.com/search?q=cache:IpstxCVYhp4J:https://impossiblefoods.com/blog/the-agonizing-dilemma-of-animal-testing&cd=11&hl=en&ct=clnk&gl=au
13. Herzog, H. (2014). 84% of Vegetarians and Vegans Return to Meat. Why? https://www.psychologytoday.com/au/blog/animals-and-us/201412/84-vegetarians-and-vegans-return-meat-why

Chapter 7

1. Foer, J.S. (2019). We Are the Weather: Saving the Planet Begins at Breakfast. https://www.amazon.com.au/We-Are-Weather-Saving-Breakfast/

References

dp/0374280002
2. Psihoyos, L. (2019). The Game Changers Documentary. https://gamechangersmovie.com/
3. Fulkerson, L. (2013). Forks Over Knives. https://www.forksoverknives.com/the-film/
4. Andersen, K. & Kuhn, K. (2017). What the Health. https://www.imdb.com/title/tt5541848/
5. Joy, M. (2011). Why We Love Dogs, Eat Pigs, and Wear Cows: An Introduction to Carnism. https://www.amazon.com/Love-Dogs-Pigs-Wear-Cows/dp/1573245054
6. Dominion. (2018). Watch Dominion (2018) - Full Documentary. https://www.dominionmovement.com/watch
7. Farm Transparency Project. (2014). Farm Transparency Project - Australian Animal Protection Charity. https://www.farmtransparency.org/
8. Anderson, K. & Kuhn, K. (2014). COWSPIRACY: The Sustainability Secret. https://www.cowspiracy.com/
9. Tabrizi, A. (2021). Seaspiracy Facts. https://www.seaspiracy.org/facts
10. Winters, E. (2022). This Is Vegan Propaganda: (And Other Lies the Meat Industry Tells You). https://www.amazon.com/This-Vegan-Propaganda-Other-Industry/dp/1785043765
11. Hill, S. (2021). The Proof Is in the Plants: How Science Shows a Plant-Based Diet Could Save Your Life. https://www.amazon.com.au/Proof-Plants-science-plant-based-planet-ebook/dp/B085ZZ21RG

Chapter 8

1. Safe Food Queensland. (2021). Spotlight on Australia's Red Meat Industry. https://www.safefood.qld.gov.au/newsroom/spotlight-on-australias-red-meat-industry/
2. The Meat & Wine Co. (2020). Why Australian Meat Is the World's Best. https://themeatandwineco.com/blog/4-reasons-australian-meat-is-the-best-in-the-world/
3. Rooke, J. (2013). Do Carnivores Need Vitamin B12 Supplements? https://baltimorepostexaminer.com/carnivores-need-vitamin-b12-supplements/2013/10/30
4. Vigen, T. (2012). Per Capita Consumption of Chicken Correlates with Total US Crude Oil Imports. http://tylervigen.com/spurious-correlations
5. Fallacy Man. (2016). The Hierarchy of Evidence: Is the Study's Design Robust? https://thelogicofscience.com/2016/01/12/the-hierarchy-of-evidence-is-the-studys-design-robust/
6. Akhtar, A. (2015). The Flaws and Human Harms of Animal Experimentation. https://www.ncbi.nlm.nih.gov/pmc/articles/PMC4594046/

Chapter 9
1. Clear, J. (n.d.). Atomic Habits Summary. https://jamesclear.com/atomic-habits-summary
2. Veganuary. (2022). Veganuary 2022 Campaign in Review. https://veganuary.com/wp-content/uploads/2022/03/Veganuary-2022-End-Of-Campaign-Report.pdf
3. Willett, W., Rockström, J., Loken, B., et al. (2019). Food in the Anthropocene: The EAT–Lancet Commission on Healthy Diets from Sustainable Food Systems. https://www.thelancet.com/journals/lancet/article/PIIS0140-6736(18)31788-4/fulltext
4. Buettner, D. & Skemp, S. (2016). Blue Zones. https://www.ncbi.nlm.nih.gov/pmc/articles/PMC6125071/
5. Ritchie, H. (2022). Dairy vs. Plant-Based Milk: What Are the Environmental Impacts? https://ourworldindata.org/environmental-impact-milks
6. FAO. (2013). Food Wastage Footprint: Impacts on Natural Resources: Summary Report. https://www.fao.org/3/i3347e/i3347e.pdf

Chapter 10
1. Carbstrong, J. (2022). How to Cope with Non-Vegan Friends & Family (a Survival Guide). https://www.youtube.com/watch?v=3C1bYm_MmV4
2. Covey, S.R. (2004). The 7 Habits of Highly Effective People: Powerful Lessons in Personal Change. https://www.franklincovey.com/the-7-habits/
3. Baxter, C.K. (2021). How to Mindfully Talk About Veganism with Friends and Family. https://mamahashermindful.com/mindfully-talk-about-veganism/
4. Ramsden, P. (2017). Vicarious Trauma, PTSD and Social Media: Does Watching Graphic Videos Cause Trauma. https://www.longdom.org/proceedings/vicarious-trauma-ptsd-and-social-media-does-watching-graphic-videos-cause-trauma-37421.html

Chapter 11
1. Winerman, L. (2005). The Mind's Mirror. https://www.apa.org/monitor/oct05/mirror
2. Mcleod, S. (2022). Operant Conditioning in Psychology: B.F. Skinner Theory. https://www.simplypsychology.org/operant-conditioning.html